Pharmacoepidemiology
Principles and Practice

Pharmacoepidemiology
Principles and Practice

Brenda Waning, MPH, RPh
Assistant Professor of Pharmacy Practice
Massachusetts College of Pharmacy and Allied
Health Sciences
BOSTON, MASSACHUSETTS

Michael Montagne, RPh, PhD
Professor of Social Pharmacy
Massachusetts College of Pharmacy and Allied
Health Sciences
BOSTON, MASSACHUSETTS

With a chapter by:
William W. McCloskey, PharmD
Associate Professor of Clinical Pharmacy
Chair, Department of Pharmacy Practice
Massachusetts College of Pharmacy and Allied
Health Sciences
BOSTON, MASSACHUSETTS

With illustrations by:
Rebecca A. Maki

McGraw-Hill
Medical Publishing Division

New York St. Louis San Francisco Auckland Bogotá Caracas
Lisbon London Madrid Mexico City Milan Montreal
New Delhi San Juan Singapore Sydney Tokyo Toronto

McGraw-Hill

*A Division of The **McGraw·Hill** Companies*

Pharmacoepidemiology: Principles and Practice

Copyright © 2001 by The **McGraw-Hill** Companies, Inc. All rights reserved. Printed in the United States of America. Except as permitted under the United States Copyright Act of 1976, no part of this publication may be reproduced or distributed in any form or by any means, or stored in a data base or retrieval system, without the prior written permission of the publisher.

1 2 3 4 5 6 7 8 9 0   DOC/DOC   0 9 8 7 6 5 4 3 2 1 0

ISBN: 0-07-135507-3

The book was set in Horley Old Style by the PRD Group.
The editor was Stephen Zollo.
The production supervisor was Clare Stanley.
Project management was provided by Spectrum Publishing Services.
The cover designer was by Aimee Nordin.
R.R. Donnelley & Sons was the printer and binder.

This book is printed on acid-free paper.

Library of Congress Cataloging-in-Publication Data

Waning, Brenda.
   Pharmacoepidemiology : principles and practice / Brenda Waning, Michael Montagne.
      p. cm.
   Includes bibliographical references.
   ISBN 0-07-135507-3
   1. Pharmacoepidemiology.   I. Montagne, Michael.   II. Title

RM302.5.W36 2001
615'.704–dc21   00-045207

To Our Parents
Richard and Ruth Waning
and
Margaret and Roland Montagne
With Love

CONTENTS

This book is designed primarily for undergraduate, professional educational experiences with students and practicing pharmacists. The concepts and methods of pharmacoepidemiology are also of value to other health professionals, public health workers, members of pharmaceutical industry, and anyone who is interested in an introductory review of pharmacoepidemiology.

Pharmacoepidemiology texts and reference books have become available recently for the graduate student in public health, medicine, and the pharmaceutical sciences. Epidemiology has not been as accessible for undergraduate and professional students. There are currently very few instances of required pharmacoepidemiology coursework in the curricula of American colleges of pharmacy. Public health courses, once required in the pharmaceutical curricula up through the 1970s, are no longer available to most student pharmacists. This makes it difficult to introduce epidemiology, the scientific method of public health, without a basis in public health. The first two chapters, then, are an attempt to provide the reader with a sense of the foundation of epidemiology in public health, through the study of populations, in which health problems are identified, assessed, and prevented or resolved.

Our experiences, and input from colleagues in pharmacy, public health, medical sociology, and statistics, have led us to believe that the best focus of our primer would be for students in research methods or drug literature evaluation courses. Our introductory review of the principles and methods of epidemiology, statistics, and their application to drug use and postmarketing surveillance of pharmaceutical products, is intended to provide a basic understanding of what pharmacoepidemiology is and how it works in practice. Along the way, readers also will be introduced briefly to public health and epidemiology. Some readers may become interested enough in this subject to pursue careers in this growing discipline. After finishing our primer, students and other readers, who desire more advanced knowledge, skills, and case studies, are strongly encouraged to pursue graduate-level and professional texts, as well as the journals, conferences, and organizations that represent pharmacoepidemiology.

We gratefully acknowledge the assistance of Rebecca Maki for wonderful illustrations, Tracy Ward for organizational assistance with the manuscript, and our very patient editor at McGraw-Hill, Steve Zollo. Brenda Waning thanks her friend and mentor, Sue Fish, for convincing her to pursue a graduate education in public health. Mike Montagne still is eternally grateful that the University of Minnesota College of Pharmacy had required public health courses in their curriculum (at least in the 1970s), and that James Anthony convinced him to be a post-doctoral fellow at Johns Hopkins University and provided, along with other faculty, an excellent foundation in epidemiology and public health.

We are interested in receiving ideas, case studies, criticisms, and suggestions from our readers. Please send them to us in care of McGraw-Hill. We hope readers enjoy and learn from our primer, and we wish them all the best in their pharmacoepidemiological investigations.

Brenda Waning
Michael Montagne
Boston, Massachusetts

Chapter 1

Introduction to Epidemiology and Public Health

On an almost daily basis, people read or hear about new drug discoveries and adverse reactions supposedly caused by drugs on the market. Sometimes panic sets in because a drug seems to be responsible for the death of some of its users, but how can people evaluate what they read and hear? How are adverse reactions and side effects studied and measured? How are a drug's beneficial effects determined? To answer these questions and many others about medications and drugs used in society, data and information are gathered and analyzed through pharmacoepidemiological study.

In this book, the principles and practice of pharmacoepidemiology are presented and discussed in the contexts of epidemiology and public health. In an attempt to prevent or reduce the occurrence of disease, public health professionals realized a scientific method was needed to assess diseases and their causes. In essence, they needed to develop a logical, standard approach to counting events (e.g. births, deaths, disease) and calculating results from the data. The field of epidemiology was born in the 19th century to address this need. In the latter half of the 20th century, epidemiologists applied the basic principles of their discipline to study the occurrence of drug use and associated problems. Thus, at the foundation of pharmacoepidemiology is epidemiology.

In this chapter, the basic aspects of epidemiology and public health are introduced as the basis for understanding pharmacoepidemiology. The host–agent–environment model is presented as the guide to comprehending disease occurrence and transmission in a population.

Epidemiology and Public Health

Whereas epidemiology is the study of disease occurrence and transmission in a human population, epidemiological studies focus on the distribution and determinants of disease. Epidemiology may also be considered the method of public health—a scientific approach to studying disease and health problems.

1

Epidemiology consists of research methods and specific strategies for counting and calculating the occurrence and risk of disease. Therefore, epidemiological studies of drug use employ these methods and statistical measures to study the occurrence and distribution of drug use and its associated problems. Examples of epidemiology applied to drug use include adverse drug reaction reporting, postmarketing surveillance studies, and clinical drug trials.

One major difference between the clinician's and the epidemiologist's perspective is the focus on individual patients versus the population at large. For example, health professionals are educated to focus on individual patient problems, and pharmacists are trained to consider individual patient variability in response to drug therapy. The focus in both of these areas in health care emphasizes interactions with individual patients. Health professionals sometimes assume that if their patient has a problem with a drug, then many other patients also have the same problem. This assumption may be flawed because the nature and extent of the problem in other patients cannot be known by these health professionals. Only by studying large groups of people (ie, populations) can the magnitude and reasons for a problem be determined.

In contrast, the public health perspective considers the population as a whole as the focus of its inquiry. Health problems are viewed as occurring in large groups of people—the population under study—and the primary goal is to measure the occurrence and development of these problems. If an individual patient is one of only a few people with a specific health problem, then the health problem would be viewed as a less significant public health concern than another situation in which a large number of people had the same condition.

Epidemiologists categorize disease and drug use primarily by time, place, and person. They try to determine whether there has been an increase or a decrease in a health problem in a specific place during a defined period. They also attempt to characterize how a disease originates, how it develops and spreads through a population, and ways to prevent or reduce its occurrence and continual harmful effects.

Epidemiologists basically count and analyze health problems in terms of proportions and rates. The history of epidemiology is a story of discovering ways of identifying and counting specific health problems.

Historical Development of Epidemiology

The development of epidemiology has spanned many centuries. Key events in the development of epidemiology include James Lind's studies on scurvy from 1747 through 1753, the standardized registration of births and deaths in the early 1800s, and John Snow's observations of a cholera epidemic in London in 1849. Although key developments in epidemiology have occurred over the past 3 centuries, the field emerged as an area of medical inquiry only in the late 19th century.

A seminal moment in the origins of epidemiology came in 1662 with the publication of John Graunt's *Natural and Political Observations, mentioned in a following index and made upon the bills of mortality.*[1] Graunt had collected London's bills of mortality, or death, as well as those of a parish town in

Hampshire, which had been initiated in 1603 by parish clerks. He organized this information and derived implications about mortality and fertility in the two populations. Graunt noted an unusual excess of male births, a high infant mortality rate, and seasonal variations in mortality. He attempted to distinguish mortality from acute causes versus chronic diseases and examined urban–rural differences in death rates. He also constructed the first known life table, a numerical representation summarizing mortality in terms of the number, percent, and probability of living or dying throughout a lifetime. Graunt also proposed that each country should develop similar tables for comparison and to construct a general law of mortality.

The first clinical drug trial, although it was not called that, took place more than 2 centuries ago. It signaled the shift from therapeutics as an art to therapeutics as a science. In 1753, James Lind published his major medical study, *A Treatise on the Scurvy*.[2] Scurvy, the condition caused by a lack of vitamin C, plagued sailors and other people who could not eat fresh fruit on a regular basis.

In Lind's study aboard a ship at sea in 1747, he identified 12 sailors with scurvy, each having similar symptoms and characteristics. He placed the sailors in one area and imposed a common diet. After some time, the sailors were divided into pairs. Each of the 6 pairs received one of the following treatments: (1) 25 drops of elixir of vitriol (copper or iron sulfate) 3 times a day on an empty stomach; (2) 2 spoonsful of vinegar 3 times a day; (3) a quart of cider each day; (4) a half pint of seawater every day; (5) a medicinal paste made of garlic, mustard, myrrh, and balsam of Peru; or (6) 2 oranges and 1 lemon daily. According to Lind's results, the most sudden, visible, beneficial effects were obtained from the use of oranges and lemons. One of the sailors who had taken the citrus fruit was fit for duty at the end of 6 days. The other sailor had the best recovery of any of the other sailors in a similar condition.

One of the first modern epidemiologists was Pierre-Charles Louis, a statistician whose work focused on the comparison of groups of people.[2] In the 1830s, he conducted several observational studies, including one that demonstrated that blood letting was an ineffective treatment. Louis pioneered the use of statistical methods in medicine.

Victorian England was one of the first societies to focus on the public health of its people. The London Epidemiological Society was formed to determine the etiology, or cause, of cholera, and included a series of classic studies on cholera by John Snow.[2] It also was involved in the study of the smallpox vaccine. Snow investigated the occurrence of cholera in London from 1848 through 1854. During that time, several water companies were responsible for supplying water to different parts of London. Snow noted that the rates of cholera were particularly high in the areas supplied by two specific companies that obtained their water from the Thames River at a point heavily polluted with sewage. From 1849 through 1854, one of the companies changed its water source to a less contaminated part of the Thames.

In 1854, another cholera epidemic occurred. Two thirds of London's population south of the Thames was served by the same two water companies. In this area, adjacent houses were receiving their water from one of the two different companies. Snow counted the number of cholera deaths in neighborhood households and matched it to their source of water. His findings were incredibly clear: The water company drawing its water from the polluted part of the Thames was associated with the highest household death rate from cholera. The company's water source was changed, and legislation began mandating that all water companies filter their water. Cholera outbreaks then declined.

Many other examples demonstrate the value of epidemiology in identifying the source and spread of disease. Epidemiology has been useful in identifying diseases caused by vitamin and mineral deficiencies; exposure to toxins and radiation; and, of course, infectious diseases caused by various organisms. Epidemiologists also study chronic diseases. The natural history of cardiovascular disease, cancer, AIDS, and various mental illnesses also have been identified and described through epidemiological inquiry.

Pharmacoepidemiology

With a recent resurgence of interest in drug epidemiology, or *pharmacoepidemiology*, has come the development of concepts and methods to assess drug use. Although pharmacoepidemiology is a relatively new term, research on drug use in epidemiology and public health has been ongoing for at least 4 decades. It is even possible to trace pharmacoepidemiological concepts back many centuries to Lind's "clinical trial" using citrus fruit to treat scurvy, which was published in 1753, and studies by William Withering on the therapeutic effects of foxglove, published in 1785.[2]

Medication use always has been important in American society, and, since the 1990s, use of prescription medications has been increasing considerably. Along with this increase in use has come more problems associated with the use of specific medications (e.g., adverse reactions, side effects). Effective medications are needed, and replacing older drugs with newer ones has been a key aspect of health care advances. Unfortunately, newer, more specific-acting drugs also have problems associated with their use.

Although the pharmaceutical profession has traditionally been involved in the preparation and distribution of drug products, great advances in drug development throughout the 20th century have shifted the focus of their work. The pharmaceutical industry has become the primary producer of finished dosage forms. By the end of the century, pharmacy had become increasingly engaged in ensuring the safe and rational use of manufactured medications. The new mission for pharmacy is to enhance society's ability to use pharmaceutical products in an optimally effective manner and, by extension, to limit or prevent the occurrence of drug use problems. To achieve this goal, pharmaceutical professionals must become skilled in developing and using concepts and methods for assessing the nature and extent of drug use.

Pharmacoepidemiology currently focuses on pharmaceutical care outcomes and the identification of potential or realized drug use problems. The discipline's basis in epidemiology provides a theoretical foundation for examining the source of supply and flow of drugs throughout a population as well as the effects experienced by individual drug users in that population. This area of research also has been used to study illicit, or nonmedical, drug use—a means to examine outbreaks of increased use called *drug epidemics*. From this perspective, drugs are viewed much like contagions or toxins, just as infectious disease epidemiology looks for the cause of epidemics or outbreaks of disease. These contagions (ie, drugs) are carried from their source, or reservoir, to their ultimate user via a variety of routes. It is important to realize that in most populations there is a relationship between the legal and the illicit drug reservoirs.

Pharmacoepidemiology in Practice

The basic idea of pharmacoepidemiology is to measure the source, diffusion, use, and effects of drugs in a population and to determine the frequency and distribution of drug use outcomes in that population. From this information, the nature and extent of specific types of drug use can be determined, and both potential and realized problems can be identified.

The focus of this type of research includes (1) what is being used (an assessment of specific drugs being used in certain situations); (2) how it is being used (an assessment of the patterns of use, including how much, where and when, and by whom); and (3) why it is being used (an assessment of the reasons for drug-taking behaviors and the functions that drugs serve in society). The latter focus on the reasons for use is rarely included in most pharmacoepidemiological studies.

The World Health Organization[3] focuses its pharmacoepidemiological efforts on ensuring the quality, safety, and efficacy of drugs and their use in specific populations. The organization's pharmacoepidemiological studies are performed to (1) describe current patterns of drug use in specific patient populations; (2) determine changes in drug use over time; (3) measure the effects of information, education, promotional activities, media accounts, and price on drug use; (4) detect inappropriate drug use and associated problems; (5) estimate drug needs in terms of disease patterns and outbreaks; and (6) plan the selection, supply, and distribution of drugs.[3]

The research methods used most often by pharmacoepidemiologists include terms familiar to readers of medical and pharmaceutical journals: the *cross-sectional study*, a prevalence survey of health and illness in the population at one point in time; the *case-control study*, a retrospective analysis comparing subjects with the condition (cases) to those without it (controls) with respect to possible risk or causative factors; and the *cohort study*, an incidence study that follows a population free of health problems over time, examining subsequent development of problems and factors associated with them. *Clinical trials*, an experimental approach that tests the value of a new treatment or intervention compared with a standard treatment or a placebo, are also considered to be an epidemiological method.

Many sources of data and information about drug-taking behaviors exist (see Table 1-1). Each source of data has its own unique advantages and limitations. Many studies report only frequencies of use without any basis in the population from which they were derived. Epidemiological measures are based on rates, with a numerator divided by a denominator. Reporting that 100 patients are experiencing an adverse reaction to a new drug (the numerator), without giving a sense of whether this effect is occurring in a population of 10,000 or 1,000,000 users of that drug (the denominator) provides only marginally useful information. This information is even more important in studying trends in drug use and determining when the risk of an adverse reaction might outweigh its beneficial effects for a patient. Denominator data are very important because, without them, comparisons are impossible.

Epidemiology aids in the discovery of benefits and hazards of drug use. For example, epidemiological research uncovered the cancer-inducing effects of estrogens and diethylstilbestrol, yet estrogens were also found to protect women from certain cancers. Aspirin use has been found to reduce the risk of recurrent cardiovascular conditions. Widely known adverse reactions discovered by epidemiological studies include phenylbutazone and chloramphenicol-associated aplastic anemia, clindamycin-associated colitis, halothane-associated jaundice, aspirin and Reye syndrome, and a rise in asthma mortality brought about by increased use of beta-agonist bronchodilator inhalers. Epidemiological methods are also used to

---

TABLE 1-1. **Sources of Data on Drug Use**

Institutional record systems and databases
    drug utilization studies
    hospital-based medical audits (inpatient)

Systemwide databases
    institutionally based reviews (outpatient)
    health insurance groups and third-party payers
    pharmaceutical organizations
    commercial vendors of marketing studies and sales data

National databases
    government-sponsored studies
    essential drug lists and inventory data
    pharmacoepidemiological surveillance systems

Field data
    records of drug dispensers, sellers, and distributors
    drug-taking behaviors of individuals and small groups

Experimental data
    clinical trial results

TABLE 1-2. **Problem Solving with Pharmacoepidemiology**

Medical drug use
  beneficial effects of drug therapy
  risks (e.g., adverse reactions, side effects) of drug therapy
  inappropriate prescribing behaviors
  patient noncompliance
  irrational self-medication practices
  poor drug use outcomes
  cost-effectiveness of drug therapy

Nonmedical drug use
  social-recreational drug use and associated problems
  acute incidents of drug toxicities (e.g., overdoses)
  chemical dependencies
  outbreaks and sources of drug epidemics

measure illegal drug use and outbreaks of misuse, such as epidemics of heroin, methamphetamine, and cocaine use.

Drug development and approval processes are greatly dependent on data and information generated through epidemiological studies. Clinical trials test the value of drugs, such as the benefits of using propranolol to treat hypertension and other cardiovascular conditions. Postmarketing surveillance detects and measures adverse drug reactions and other unintended effects after a drug product has been released to the marketplace. Relatively new efforts have been studying the benefits and costs of drug use in economic terms (pharmacoeconomics) and in terms of patient-centered care employing quality-of-life indicators.

The future of pharmacoepidemiological studies has unlimited potential. This field represents the primary scientific approach for the pharmaceutical profession's new mission in patient care. Its approaches and techniques for assessing the nature and extent of drug use and the reasons behind unsafe or irrational use will allow the development of strategies to prevent or limit drug use problems (see Table 1-2). With these tools, the products of drug development can be used more effectively, while minimizing problems, for the benefit of both individual patients and society.

Host–Agent–Environment Model of Public Health

The core perspective of public health is the host–agent–environment model, and it is essential for understanding the rationale behind epidemiology (Figure 1-1).

The host–agent–environment model is also central to the reasoning of public health. The *host* is the recipient of the causative agent of a disease or a health problem. The *agent* is the cause of the disease, also called the contagion. (Risk

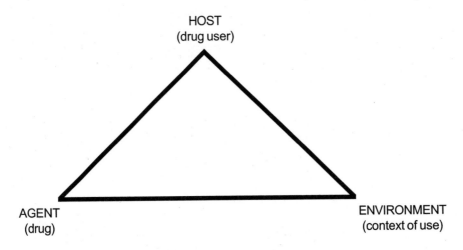

Figure 1-1. Host–agent–environment model.

factors can also be considered in this category.) The *environment* consists of the conditions affecting survival and transmission of the causative agent. The host–agent–environment model describes how these three main factors interrelate to bring about disease.

When public health professionals classify agent, host, and environmental factors that determine the occurrence of diseases in human populations, they include agents of disease, also called etiological factors; host factors, also called intrinsic factors; and environmental factors, also called extrinsic factors.

For this discussion, the host is typically a human being; and aspects such as exposures, susceptibility, response to agents, and general human characteristics and behaviors all comprise the intrinsic factors. Host, or intrinsic, factors include genetics (e.g., sickle-cell disease), age (e.g., Alzheimer's disease), gender (e.g., rheumatoid arthritis), ethnic group, physiological state, prior immunological experience, current or preexisting diseases, and human behavior. With regard to human behavior, epidemiologists study personal hygiene, food handling, diet, interpersonal contacts, occupation, recreation, use of health resources, tobacco and alcohol use, and a wide range of complex behaviors.

Agents of disease, or etiological factors, can consist of many things beyond infectious diseases. Excesses or deficiencies in nutritional elements, exposure to chemical agents (e.g., drugs, poisons, allergens), and contact with physical agents all may play a role in bringing about the occurrence of a specific disease. Examples of etiological factors include excesses of cholesterol; common deficiencies of vitamins and proteins; ragweed and poison ivy; and, of course, a range of infectious agents, such as protozoa, bacteria, fungi, and viruses.

Environmental, or extrinsic, factors influence the existence of the agent as well as exposure or susceptibility to the agent. These factors may include the physical environment (e.g., geology, climate), the biological environment (e.g., human populations, flora, fauna), and the socioeconomic environment (e.g., occupations, urbanization, economic development, disruptions from wars and natural disasters).

Disease Occurrence and Transmission

An outbreak of a disease, also called an *epidemic,* is a sudden, dramatic increase in the number of people with the condition or health problem. It is usually defined in terms of a specific population in a geographic area during some period. The first case indicating the possible occurrence of a disease—in other words, the first person exhibiting the signs and symptoms of the disease—marks the onset of the disease outbreak.

Each person exhibiting the signs and symptoms of the disease may have a different time of onset compared with another person, but a distribution of the times of individual disease onsets can be constructed as an epidemic curve. An *incubation period* is the interval of time between exposure to, or contact with, the causative agent (or risk factor) and the onset of the condition. Individuals have their own incubation periods, whereas an epidemic has its specific incubation period, which can be identified as the median case on the epidemic curve. The epidemic curve for a specific disease is fairly consistent from outbreak to outbreak, and it becomes a distinguishing feature of that disease.

Human disease is classified by selected epidemiological features. Disease is transmitted from host to host though a specific mechanism. The causative agent invades the body through a portal of entry and may exit from that same portal or a different place. The portal of entry or exit in the human host can include the upper respiratory tract (e.g., diphtheria), the lower respiratory tract (e.g., tuberculosis), the gastrointestinal tract (e.g., typhoid), the genital-urinary tract (e.g., gonorrhea), or through the eyes, skin, or other tissues.

The dynamics of the spread of a disease include the reservoirs, where the agent may reside; vectors (living things), and vehicles (inanimate objects) that aid in the transmission or spread of the causative agent; and cycles in the natural history of the disease. The principal reservoirs of infection include humans and other vertebrates; some causative agents are able to live free of a host. Examples of common vehicles are food, water, air, and inoculation. Propagation of disease by serial transfer from host to host may occur through the respiratory, oral, anal, or genital route. Cycles of infectious agent transmission in nature include human to human, human to arthropod to human, vertebrate to vertebrate to human, and other combinations.

Disease Causation and Manifestation

Not every host, or human being, who is exposed to the contagion or causative agent of a disease will develop the symptoms of that disease. In other words, although every member of a defined population may have been exposed to a causative agent, not everyone will develop the disease. Many factors can mitigate the impact of a disease-causing agent, including degree of exposure, individual immune response, past exposure and experience with the agent, other medical conditions or drug therapies that are present, and even the effects of unintended treatments (through the treatment of other conditions that might mask the presence of the disease or its symptoms).

The most important issue is that of disease causation versus its manifestation; that is, whether the symptoms are of the disease itself, the body's response to the disease, or an indirect result of the disease process.

Etiology of Disease

One of the primary purposes of epidemiology is to discover the etiology, the cause or the source, of a specific disease or a group of diseases. One example of the use of epidemiological data to determine specific etiological factors is the investigation of an outbreak of food poisoning to determine which food was contaminated with the microorganism responsible for the epidemic. Another example is the study of a disease that occurs with higher frequency among workers in occupations exposing them to particular chemicals, as illustrated in a study of asbestos and cancer.

On occasion, investigators find that the increased exposure of individuals to certain agents results in a decreased frequency of a disease. A classic example of this kind of relationship is that between the presence of fluoride in the water supply and dental caries.

Investigators also attempt to determine whether an etiological hypothesis developed clinically, experimentally, or from other epidemiological studies is consistent with the epidemiological characteristics of the disease in the human population. Many studies of the relationship between oral contraceptive use and various forms of cardiovascular disease illustrate this approach. Over many years, epidemiological studies have shown a relationship between oral contraceptive use and thromboembolic disease, such as stroke. This investigation began after the first in a series of case reports associated oral contraceptive use with myocardial infarction. This anecdotal information stimulated several investigators to conduct epidemiological studies of the relationship between oral contraceptive use and various cardiovascular diseases.

Discovering the etiology of a disease creates an excellent basis for preventive and public health services. It also assists in the discovery of ways to treat the condition or disease. Clinicians apply epidemiological principles in making diagnostic and therapeutic decisions, performing research, and interpreting the literature.

Drug Epidemics

Epidemiology can also be used to study illicit drug use, such as outbreaks of heroin, cocaine, or amphetamine use and other drug use problems. As depicted in Figure 1-2, drug use problems are viewed as public health concerns.[4]

Several concepts from communicable-disease epidemiology are helpful in defining the source of supply and flow of drugs through a population. Drugs are

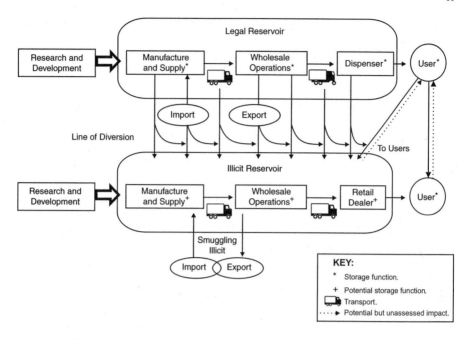

Figure 1-2. Host–agent–environment model applied to drug use.[4]

viewed as analogous to microbial agents in the communicable-disease model. Thus, the reservoir for drugs may be defined roughly as the means by which the drug becomes available for consumption and through which availability is sustained.

The upper half of Figure 1-1 represents the legally authorized channels of drug research and development, supply, and distribution to authorized consumers of a drug product. The open arrow between the drug research and development units, and the supply and manufacturing units, illustrates that there is relatively little flow of drug product between these units. The flow is primarily one of ideas and techniques.

In this representation, supply of the drug begins with the succession of manufacturing and importation and proceeds to wholesale distribution and other storage locations. The figure shows distribution flowing from the wholesale unit to retail units (e.g., pharmacy, clinic), where a drug is stored until it is dispensed to an authorized consumer, who may dispose of it at once or keep it stored and release it over time.

Some of the legally imported and manufactured drug supplies move through authorized channels of distribution to unauthorized consumers or move directly from an authorized consumer to an unauthorized consumer. This diversion (shown by means of arrows crossing a line of diversion) may occur throughout the reservoir, with or without the cooperation of the authorized manufacturer, wholesaler, prescriber, or consumer. Unauthorized channels of drug research and development, supply, and distribution are represented in the bottom half of the figure. The possibility for unauthorized supply through bootlegging and smuggling also is represented in the lower half of the figure. Diversion from authorized wholesalers and dispensers and from authorized common carriers that transport the drug product is also possible.

In this figure, drug distributors, prescribers, dispensers, and consumers are included as elements of the drug reservoir. Consumers are included because they may be means of drug availability to other people. Consumers also might be regarded as vectors, carrying batches of the drug away from the manufacturer or dispenser toward ultimate consumers. Either view is compatible with the development of epidemiological ideas on drug use and drug use problems.

It is important to notice the involvement of inanimate objects or materials in the storage and conveyance of drugs to and from the reservoir. These include screened and locked areas within factories, containers for shipping between factories and distributors, unit-dose or other pill containers in which medicines are dispensed, and other ingredients in the formulation of the drug product. Viewing the pill containers, fillers, and other materials as vehicles draws attention to them as modifiable aspects of agent transmission to a host. Once a drug reaches the ultimate consumer and is ingested, there begins an interaction of this drug agent, the human host, and the environment. The results of human exposure to a drug agent cannot be understood fully without consideration of this interaction.

In the 1960s and 1970s, epidemiologists applied the host–agent–environment model to study epidemics of heroin use. Illicit drug use was viewed as a practice that was transmitted from one person to another, like a type of contagious illness. This approach made it possible to apply the methods and terminology of infectious disease epidemiology to the study of illicit drug use.

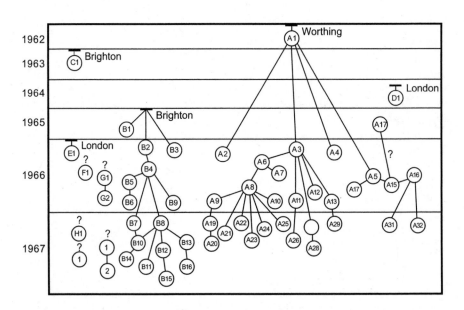

Figure 1-3. Heroin epidemic in Crawley, England in 1967.
The United Nations is the author of the original material.

In 1967, in the small town of Crawley, England, there was a sudden and dramatic increase in the number of heroin users.[5] Heroin addicts identified by the psychiatric service were interviewed regarding their first injection of heroin and with whom they socialized (see Figure 1-3). The analysis of this heroin epidemic followed the classic epidemiological framework of identifying an onset, environment, agent (which was heroin), mode of transmission, and source of contagion (initial users).

A high prevalence of heroin use was found in Crawley in 1967. Yearly incidence rates were calculated, and the source of the contagion was identified. Three stages in the spread of heroin in Crawley emerged: (1) from 1962 through 1965, a small number of Crawley teens (virtually all males) were initiated into heroin use in nearby towns; (2) during the first half of 1966, a nucleus of established heroin users initiated by the former (first wave of) users developed in Crawley; and (3) from the latter half of 1966 through the first half of 1967, heroin use spread quickly in Crawley to reach the "epidemic" proportions that initiated the retrospective study in late 1967. Forty-eight individual heroin users were traced back along 2 primary transmission trees (routes) to 2 single sources. This study helped the residents of Crawley to plan treatment and prevention activities to fight the heroin epidemic.

Summary

In the public health perspective, epidemiology is the primary approach for identifying and describing the occurrence and development of disease. It also is useful in identifying the nature and extent of drug use as well as problems resulting from the use of drugs. The public health model and epidemiological methods provide a means for measuring, analyzing, and interpreting patterns of drug use and associated problems in society. In this chapter, the basic foundation of epidemiology and public health was presented along with a brief historical review and the application of epidemiology to the study of drug use and its effects—pharmacoepidemiology—were described.

References

1. Vogt DD, Montagne M. The process of drug development: II. The historical interplay of therapeutics, clinical research, and scientific education. *Clin Res Practices & Drug Regul Affairs*. 1983; 1:177–201.

2. Clendening L, ed. *Source Book of Medical History*. New York, NY: Dover, 1960.

3. World Health Organization. *The Rational Use of Drugs*. Geneva: Author; 1987.

4. Anthony, JC. The regulation of dangerous psychoactive drugs. In: Morgan JP, Kagan DV, eds. *Society and Medication: Conflicting Signals for Prescribers and Patients*. Lexington, Mass: DC Health Co.; 1983; 163–180.

5. DeAlarcon R. The spread of heroin abuse in a community. *Bull Narcot*. 1969; 21:17–22.

Study Questions

1. What is the primary difference in the focus of inquiry between clinical medicine and epidemiology?

2. Who performed the first clinical drug trial in history, and how was the study performed?

3. Briefly describe the importance of each component in the host–agent–environment model as it relates to the occurrence and transmission of a disease.

4. Define the following terms:

    a. onset

    b. etiology

    c. vehicle

    d. vector

    e. portal of entry or exit

    f. reservoir

    g. mode of transmission

    h. epidemic

    i. incubation period

    j. epidemiology

    k. pharmacoepidemiology

5. A *Boston Globe* article published in late 1997 reported that Seldane® was considered to be unsafe by the U.S. Food and Drug Administration. The article suggested that Seldane® should be removed from the market. The *Globe* reported that since the drug's introduction in 1985 it has been blamed for perhaps hundreds of deaths from unstable heart rhythms when taken with the common antibiotic erythromycin. Patients with liver disease have also reported abnormal heart rhythms when taking Seldane® alone. According to the *Globe*, pharmacists filled 6.5 million prescriptions for Seldane® during 1997. What does it mean to say that hundreds of deaths make the drug unsafe?

    a. Did the *Globe* article provide a denominator to give a sense of how many people were taking Seldane® and, thus, what proportion of the population using this drug might be susceptible to the dangerous side effects?

    b. Was any type of denominator provided in the *Globe* article that might be useful in calculating a proportion or a rate of occurrence for the problem?

    c. If the specific number of deaths was 200, then what would the death rate be per 100,000 prescriptions?

    d. If the specific number of deaths was 2000, then what would the death rate be per 100,000 prescriptions?

6. In July 1998, consumer advocacy groups urged the government to ban a new diabetes drug that was widely promoted as a way to help some patients reduce their need for insulin shots. The call to ban Rezulin® came 7 months after the drug was pulled off the market in Great Britain because of potential liver injury. The U.S. Food and Drug Administration responded that Rezulin® offers an important benefit for type II diabetics who are not adequately helped by other drugs. The *Boston Globe* reported that in the first 15 months the drug was available on the market, 26 deaths from liver failure had been reported worldwide among users of this drug, 100 people had been hospitalized for liver toxicity, and 3 liver transplants had been done. A "Dear Doctor" letter was sent from the manufacturer, Parke-Davis, to 500,000 physicians warning them about this potential adverse reaction.

a. Are 26 deaths from liver failure sufficient reason (number) to warrant removal of this drug product from the market?

b. Was any denominator information provided in this story?

c. Assume that 650,000 prescriptions were written for Rezulin in the first 15 months it was on the market. During that same period, what was the death rate per 100,000 prescriptions?

Chapter 2

Medical Surveillance and Outbreaks of Disease

One of the initial reasons for developing epidemiological concepts and methods was to study the natural history of disease. With knowledge about the cause(s) of a disease or health problem, a solution could be derived, along with preventive measures for the future. The two primary intents were to identify, describe, and understand infectious disease epidemics that could kill a large part of a population and to maintain health surveillance of a population so that new diseases and problems could be recognized.

Surveillance continues to be a very important aspect of public health. It is the central function of pharmacoepidemiology, as noted, for instance, in the postmarketing surveillance of pharmaceutical products. The goal of this activity is identification of adverse reactions, side effects, and even new beneficial effects of medications used by a population.

Medical Surveillance

One of the most basic functions of epidemiology is detecting the occurrence of health problems or exposures in a target population. This process of detection, called *medical surveillance,* is conducted to identify changes in the distribution of diseases, thereby permitting their prevention or control within the population. The term *surveillance* means "to watch over." Medical surveillance traditionally involved monitoring the spread of infectious diseases through a population. Today, however, surveillance programs are applied to a variety of health problems and conditions. Medical surveillance involves the following key features:

- Continuous data collection and evaluation
- An identified target population
- A standard definition of the outcome under study
- Timely collection and dissemination of information
- Application of the data to disease control and prevention

Surveillance activities provide data about the distribution of a disease by person, place, and time. These three classic variables are the most important in epidemiology, because patterns of occurrence indicated by these variables can help identify possible causes of a disease. A great variety of information is collected during surveillance, including demographic information about affected and unaffected individuals, their behaviors, and the geographic location of health problems.

Many diseases, such as cancer, heart conditions, sexually transmitted diseases, and drug addiction, are studied through medical surveillance. The goals of medical surveillance activities include the following:

- Identifying patterns of disease occurrence
- Detecting disease outbreaks or epidemics
- Developing ideas about possible causes
- Identifying cases for further investigation
- Planning health services to fulfill specific needs

The term *population-based* means that the target group under study or surveillance is the general population, usually in terms of geographic residence.

Counting in Epidemiology: Rates and Proportions

The key aspect of medical surveillance, and epidemiology as a method, is the notion of counting. Numerical results compiled in various formats represent the information available to epidemiologists for deriving answers to research questions.

Some of the terms used to represent numerical findings in epidemiology can be confusing. Good examples of often-misused terms include ratio, proportion, percentage, and rate. In general, a *ratio* is the relation in number, degree, or quantity that exists between two items, such as variables or factors. The relationship is fixed in number or degree and applies to 2 similar items, such as 50 males to 25 females, for a ratio of 2 males to 1 female (also expressed as 2 : 1). In a mathematical sense, a ratio is a result of one quantity divided by another quantity of the same kind, and it is often expressed as a fraction. Ratios are less useful than rates in descriptive statistics, and ratios are of even less value in inferential statistics.

Whereas a ratio is a general type of measure, rate, proportion, and percentage are more specific examples. In a ratio, the numerator is not included in the population defined by the denominator. No restrictions exist on the range or dimension of a ratio. There are, however, limitations on rates, proportions, percentages, incidence rates, and other epidemiological measures, for instance, in terms of the range of possible values. Ratios have been expressed as percentages in epidemiology, resulting in some confusion. All rates can be viewed as ratios, but ratios are not necessarily rates.

A proportion is a type of ratio, and a percentage is a type of proportion. A *proportion* is a relation between the amount, number, size, or degree of one item and the amount, number, size, or degree of another item. A proportion is basically a ratio whose numerator is contained in its denominator. In epidemiology, if the number of people who currently have a disease or condition is expressed relative to the total number of people who could have the disease or condition, then this ratio is referred to as a proportion. In the strictest sense of the definition, a proportion must fall within the range of 0 to 1.0.

A *percentage* is a number in each 100 of something. The word *percent* means "per 100." A proportion multiplied by 100 will produce a percent. A proportion, or a rate, also may be multiplied by a larger number, usually to make the final number more manageable or understandable for making comparisons. This number is expressed in terms of the larger number by which it was multiplied. For example, if 2 people from a group of 5000 people have a specific health problem, then the proportion of people with that problem would be expressed numerically as 2/5000, or 0.0004. This number is unmanageable for reporting and conceptualizing in relation to human beings. By multiplying this proportion by 10,000, the numerical expression becomes 4 (people) per 10,000 (population), which has the same mathematical value as 0.0004 but is easier to comprehend and use.

A *rate* is the number of one item measured in relation to units of another item. A rate can be the measure (the number or frequency) of an event, condition, injury, disability, or death per unit size of a population during a specified period. Three numbers are needed to calculate a rate: the numerator (which consists of the number of individuals affected or ill); the denominator (the total population of a specific area under study, of which the cases in the numerator are a part or from which the cases are derived), and the specific time period of the investigation (a 1-year timeframe is most commonly used).

Rates are usually presented as fractions. The result is sometimes multiplied by 100, 1000, or another basic number (usually a multiple of 10) to complete the rate and to make it more manageable. The numerator is confined to a specific set of characteristics, as defined by the study, and the denominator is limited to the study's target population. There are three general types of rates: crude rates, specific rates, and adjusted rates. All of these will be discussed later. A rate can be considered to be "true" only if the numerator is included as part of the count of the denominator and if the denominator represents the entire population of concern or the entire population at risk.

High rates, low rates, and changes in rates provide useful information and insight into the cause, spread, transmission, and overall impact of a disease on a population. Using rates, groups of healthy people can be compared with groups of ill people living in the same area. Information about rates of diseases is very useful to public health professionals who develop control or prevention programs.

Morbidity and Mortality

Morbidity and mortality are two very important aspects of medical surveillance. They are primary indicators of the healthiness or sickness of a population.

Any disturbance in the function or structure of a human body is considered to be a *disease*. Disease, illness, injury, disorder, and sickness all are categorized under a single term, morbidity. *Morbidity* is the extent of disease, illness, injury, or disability in a defined population. It is either a deviation from a state of health and well-being or the presence of a specific symptom or condition. Morbidity is usually expressed in terms of prevalence, attack rates, or incidence rates. In essence, morbidity refers to the rate of disease in a population—in other words, the number of ill people present in a certain population that is healthy but at risk for developing the disease.

Mortality means death, or it describes death and related issues. The mortality rate is the rapidity with which people in a given population die of a particular condition. Three things generally cause death: degeneration of vital organs and related conditions; specific disease states; and massive trauma or physical harm caused by environmental or social conditions, such as accidents, disasters, and homicides.

Numerical information about death is a basic component of vital statistics and epidemiology. In many countries, laws require the registration of vital events, including births, marriages, divorces, and deaths. Mortality rates are the foundation for vital statistics. Deaths are certified by a physician or a coroner; they must be recorded and reported to local health departments or state offices of vital statistics. On a death certificate, the cause of death is stated, or an underlying cause of death can be noted.

Mortality statistics are reported from the information recorded on death certificates. Public health agencies and other organizations (e.g., insurance companies) produce and revise tables of mortality that are published on a regular basis. These tables of mortality provide actual numbers of deaths as well as death rates by age, sex, and cause of death. Special mortality tables can also present other variables in the context of vital statistics. Examples of different types of mortality rates include annual death rate, infant mortality rate, fetal death rate, abortion rate, maternal mortality rate, and case fatality rate.

The mortality rate, or death rate, describes the frequency of deaths in a group or population during a given timeframe.

Mortality (death) rate (MR): rapidity with which people in a given population die from a particular condition.

$$MR = \frac{\text{number of people who died in a population}}{\text{total number of people in that population}} \text{ per unit of time}$$

Cumulative mortality is the risk of dying during a specified period. It is the summation of mortality rates for individual time periods. Mortality rates may be expressed in person-time units, summing the number of observational years for each person being recorded. (Person-time units are described in detail later.)

Prevalence and Incidence

As a measure of morbidity, *prevalence* is the number of existing cases of a disease or condition present in a defined population at one particular point in time. Prevalence also may be viewed as the probability that a condition exists in a specific population. It is the probability of the occurrence of a condition, and it is sometimes called *point prevalence*. Throughout this book, however, only the term prevalence will be used. Prevalence and the information it provides are useful in planning public health services and medical services as well as projecting health care system needs.

Prevalence (P): probability that a condition exists in a specific population; probability of the occurrence of a condition.

$$P = \frac{\text{number of existing cases in a population}}{\text{total number of people in that population}}$$

Period prevalence is the probability of occurrence, or the total number of individuals with the condition or disease, during a specified period, instead of at one point in time. The counting of cases to determine period prevalence starts at one point in time and stops at another point in time, such as over 1 year. Period prevalence is related to point prevalence and incidence. For instance, the period prevalence for a 1-year time period is equal to the point prevalence (on the first day of the year) plus the annual incidence for that same 1-year period.

Period prevalence (PP): probability of occurrence of a condition during a specified period.

$$PP = \frac{\text{number of people with disease during time period}}{\text{total number of people in that population}}$$

Prevalence assesses the total number of people in a group or population who have a disease at a specific time. Prevalence is controlled by two elements: the number of individuals who have had the disease in the past and the length or duration of the disease. Prevalence varies in direct relation to both incidence and duration. In many instances, prevalence is equal to the incidence multiplied by the average duration of the condition.

Several factors can affect prevalence. As a new disease develops in a given population, as new cases arise, and as incidence increases, prevalence also increases. Disease duration also affects prevalence. When a disease has a longer duration, prevalence remains higher for a longer time. Intervention and treatment also affect prevalence. As treatment reduces the number of cases, the duration of the disease and the number of cases decrease—thus prevalence decreases. Prevention programs, such as immunization, prevent new cases from occurring and reduce prevalence. Prolongation of life in chronic diseases or untreated cases can increase the duration and add to the prevalence.

In summary, prevalence increases with the addition of diseased people or the subtraction of healthy people, the addition of susceptible cases or those with potential to become cases, a rise in the occurrence of new cases, or a prolongation of life among current cases. Prevalence decreases with the addition of healthy

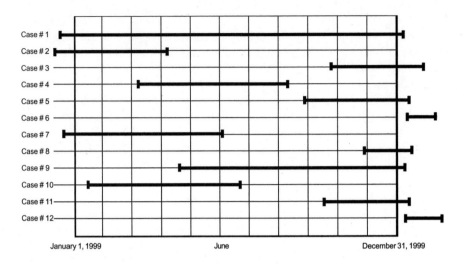

Figure 2-1. Identification of prevalence and incidence cases.

people or the deletion of sick people, improvements in cure rates, increased death rates in the diseased group, a decrease in occurrence of new cases, or a shorter duration of disease.

To practice identifying and counting specific cases while performing a prevalence calculation, consider the graph in Figure 2-1.

Figure 2-1 reveals that 10 cases of a disease in a total population of 100 people were identified as beginning, developing, or ending during a certain time period, January 1, 1999, through December 31, 1999. In addition, 2 more cases (#6, #12) were identified after the defined study period (after December 31, 1999). The length of each line in the illustration corresponds to the duration of each case (and the bar at the beginning of each solid line designates when that person's disease was diagnosed; i.e., when that person became a case). The bar at the end of each line indicates when the disease was resolved.

To calculate prevalence (point) on January 1, 3 cases would be identified and counted: cases #1, #2, and #7. Prevalence would be 3 divided by 100, which equals 0.03, multiplied by 100 (for a percent) to produce a prevalence of 3%. To calculate prevalence on December 31, 6 cases would be identified as existing on that date: cases #1, #3, #5, #8, #9, and #11. Prevalence on that date would be calculated as 6 divided by 100, to equal 0.06, which would be multiplied by 100 to produce a prevalence of 6%. The occurrence (prevalence) of this disease increased in this population during 1999. To calculate the period prevalence for 1999, the following 10 cases would be identified as existing during the 1-year timeframe: cases #1, #2, #3, #4, #5, #7, #8, #9, #10, and #11. Calculation of period prevalence would be 10 divided by 100, which equals 0.1 multiplied by 100 to produce a period prevalence for 1999 of 10%.

The *incidence rate* is a measure of the rapidity with which a new condition develops in a population. It is the rate at which the condition develops or the rate at which newly diagnosed patients are identified over time. Incidence is a bit like a motion picture, portraying the development of a disease in a population over time. Using a similar analogy, prevalence is more like a snapshot of disease present in a population at a given point in time.

Incidence rate (IR): measure of rapidity with which a new condition develops in a population; rate at which newly diagnosed patients are identified over time, measured by actural observation time.

$$IR = \frac{\text{number of new cases}}{\text{total person-time of observation in population at risk}}$$

In real-life application of incidence rates to disease outbreaks, it is often challenging to determine incidence, as the time of onset of the outbreak may be unclear. Time of diagnosis, data reporting, time of appearance of symptoms, a visit to a physician, presentation at an emergency room, or other time elements are needed to identify when an outbreak began. Incidence is not the onset of the outbreak, however, but the frequency of new cases over a time period and in a specified population.

The denominator used in calculating incidence rates should accurately describe the number at risk or under study in the group or population. The denominator consists of the individuals to whom the event may occur—in other words, the population at risk for coming down with the problem. The population may be restricted. For example, if we want to measure the incidence of recurrence or deaths after a myocardial infarction (MI), then the denominator consists only of people who have had an MI. As time passes, the number of people at risk in a population changes. Incidence rates are used to study new cases of a disease, so only individuals at risk for developing the disease should be included in the denominator. The denominator should not include individuals who already have the disease, those who have had the disease and are no longer susceptible, or those not susceptible due to intervention, such as immunization.

To determine the incidence of a disease, a group or population must be studied, specifically to ascertain the extent and rate at which new cases of the disease are occurring. When an outbreak is suspected, it is important to confirm the diagnosis of the disease or, if it is nonpathogenic in origin, to establish the source of the occurrence of an event. From this information, individuals can be classified as either diseased or not diseased. This type of information may come from self-reports or medical records.

Incidence is a rate that is expressed as a change in something per unit of time. Essential to determining incidence is time, the date of onset, or the date of disease discovery. When time of onset is difficult to determine, the most objective, clear, and earliest verifiable event must be used as the time of onset. In diseases that develop silently, such as cancer, the earliest verifiable event or diagnostic indicator is used. It is, therefore, very important to define what is meant by the onset of a condition in making calculations of incidence. When the time period of a disease under study spans an epidemic or an outbreak of very short duration, it is called an *attack rate*. (Attack rates are discussed later in this chapter.)

An incidence rate can be used to estimate the probability, or risk, of developing a disease during a specified timeframe. As the incidence rate increases, the risk or probability of contracting the disease also rises. If the incidence rate is consistently higher during a specified time of year, such as winter, then the risk of developing that disease increases during that time. If the incidence rate is consistently higher among people who live in a certain place, then the risk is higher for developing a disease if one lives in or moves to that area. If the incidence rate is consistently higher among individuals with a specific lifestyle factor, then the risk increases among the group with that lifestyle.

Incidence rates are calculated in different ways. The usual method focuses on a geographic area or place with a changing population (i.e., where there are births, deaths, immigration, and emigration). In this approach, the number of events counted during a specified period of time is divided by the average population size during that time period.

Consider Figure 2-1. In this example, incidence would be calculated by identifying all of the new cases occurring during that 1-year period, January 1 through December 31, 1999. Seven cases, #3, #4, #5, #8, #9, #10, and #11 would be labeled as the newly occurring cases. Incidence would be calculated with the numerator of 7, but the denominator would *not* be 100, the original number of people in the group. Three people (cases #1, #2, and #7) had already been diagnosed and become cases before the 1-year timeframe began—before January 1, 1999. Those 3 people were not at risk for developing the disease during 1999 because they already had the disease when the year started. As a result, these 3 people would be subtracted from the total group of 100, and the resulting denominator, 97, would be used to calculate incidence. In this example, 7 new cases would be divided by 97 to give 0.072. Multiplying this incidence rate by 100 would produce an incidence rate of 7.2%. Note that the point prevalence on January 1, 1999, was 3%, and the incidence for 1999 was 7.2%. When the point prevalence and incidence rate are added together, the result (10.2%) approximates the period prevalence (10%) for the 1-year period.

Cumulative incidence is the probability of developing a condition within a specified period. It also can be viewed as a measure of risk. The cumulative incidence rate is useful in prospective and longitudinal studies. Rates may change over time. The longer the timeframe used, the more likely it is that one could mistakenly average different rates. The cumulative incidence rate is used to study a group of people followed over the same timeframe.

Cumulative incidence: probability of developing a condition within a specified period.

In a prospective study, in which all members of a group are followed over the same time period, the incidence rate can be calculated by dividing the number of cases by the number of people in the group at the outset of the study. In a follow-up study performed on a group that contained 2000 people initially free of the disease, 100 new cases of the disease were identified during a 5-year follow-up period. The 5-year incidence rate, then, was 100 divided by 2000, or 5%. This may be called a *cumulative incidence rate* because the numerator is the number of new cases that accumulated during a defined period. It is a measure of an individual's risk of contracting the disease during this timeframe. Sometimes the term is used without the word rate and is called *cumulative incidence* or *risk*.

Another measure of incidence uses person-time units. This measure of incidence is used in studies in which individuals are at risk or observed during different time periods. Members of a group may no longer be involved in a study; they may move away, refuse to cooperate, become lost to follow up, die, or no longer be at risk. Individuals may also enter a study group at different times. For instance, any hospital-based study in which subjects are entered into the study immediately after a significant health event would produce a study group consisting of individuals observed over different timeframes.

For these reasons, incidence is often measured and reported in terms of person-time units. In a prospective study, for example, investigators track cases forward in time. When time variation is caused by individuals entering or leaving the study at different times or different ages, resulting calculations are more complex. For each individual person or case in the study, the unit of time in which she or he participated, was exposed, or was observed is used. An incidence rate with person-time units is calculated by dividing the total number of cases by the sum of the time periods relevant for each subject in the study. The length of time from a starting point through a closing point must be determined. For instance, a period of risk is defined as the length of time from being assessed to the time of either being diagnosed or withdrawing from the study or until the study ends.

Incidence rate in person-time units: incidence rate measured in person-time units due to individuals being at risk or observed for different time periods during the study; the sum of observation time periods during which individuals are at risk for all people in the study.

Person-time units make it possible to show in one number the periods of time that are used for calculation when a number of people are exposed to the same risk at various times. When sample sizes are large, risk is low, and the time period is long, person-time units work best. For person-time units to have validity and applicability, two conditions must exist. First, the probability or risk of disease must be constant throughout the entire study period. It is also assumed that those who drop out will have the same level of pathology as those who remain in and complete the study.

Consider the calculation of person-time units in Figure 2-2. In the upper diagram in this example, 10 subjects were studied for disease occurrence from January 1, 1995, through December 31, 1999. The solid line indicates the length of time a subject was observed while he or she was at risk for developing the disease. A solid square block indicates that the person was diagnosed with the disease. The broken line indicates the length of time a subject, or patient, was observed after diagnosis. The solid circle indicates that the patient died. Two patients were lost to

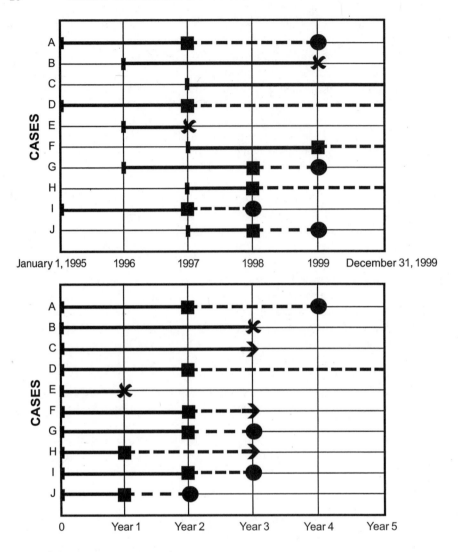

Figure 2-2. Example of incidence in person-time units.
(● = Death; x = Lost; ■ = Diagnosis.)

follow-up after a period of time. To make it easier to interpret this information and to see individual person-time units, consider the lower diagram in Figure 2-2. The data from the upper diagram have been realigned along a timeline in 1-year units, thereby allowing all 10 subjects to be compared from a base time of 0.

Subject A was observed for 2 years, then diagnosed with the disease, and observed for 2 more years until the time of death. Therefore, subject A contributed 2 person-years to the study before diagnosis. Subjects B and C each contributed

3 person-years to the study, although subject B was then lost to follow-up. Subject D contributed 2 person-years before being diagnosed. Subject E contributed 1 person-year before being lost to follow-up. Subjects F, G, and I each contributed 2 person-years, and subjects H and J each contributed 1 person-year to the study. Summing all of the person-years yields a total for the 10 subjects of 19 person-years. Calculation of incidence in this example, then, would consist of 7 (new cases during the 5-year study) divided by 19 (person-years) to equal an incidence rate of 0.37 cases/person-year, or 3.7 cases/10 person-years.

Fatality and Survival

Case fatality and survival represent mutually exclusive outcomes from being diagnosed with a disease and, together, must account for all individuals affected with the disease.

Case fatality rate (CFR): proportion of people with a particular condition who die from it in a specified time period.

$$CFR = \frac{\text{number of people who died from particular condition}}{\text{total number of people with condition}} \text{ per unit of time}$$

Survival rate (SR): likelihood of living for a specified time period after the diagnosis of a particular condition.

In the example presented in Figure 2-2, the incidence of disease has already been determined to be 3.7 cases/10 person-years. Of the 7 people who developed the disease, 4 people died from it. The case fatality rate over the 5 years of the study, then, is calculated as follows:

$$CFR = \frac{4}{7} \times 100 = 57\%$$

The survival rate is the opposite of case fatality rate. In this example, the survival rate is calculated as follows:

$$SR = 7 - \frac{4}{7} = \frac{3}{7} \times 100 = 43\%$$

Adjustments of Rates

Three types of rate are in general use. Rates used to present data or information for a total population are called *crude rates*. Any rate that conveys information or data about a population subgroup is known as a *specific rate*. This approach is used for calculating summary rates for different subgroups in a population, in which underlying differences in the distribution of a specific variable (e.g., age) are removed, thus giving rates for each specific subgroup. This calculation allows for overall comparison of two or more subgroups in a population with background differences in the distribution of specific variables. Mathematical adjustments of crude rates provide *adjusted rates*. Rates can be adjusted for age or other variables, and this approach is different from specific rates.

Crude rates are based on the number of experiences or events that happen in a total population over a certain timeframe. Vital statistics and related information are usually derived from crude rates using an average population as the denominator for each factor of population statistics. Unique differences, characteristics, behaviors, risks, and other implications for subgroups in a population are not reflected in crude rates.

Crude rates are presented not as percentages but as a rate per unit of 10 (e.g., 100,000) in a population. Crude rates are summary rates and are developed from only minimal data and limited information. For comparative purposes, they usually are valuable only in making comparisons across countries. Crude rates do not consider information derived from subgroups in special circumstances, and they fail to show differences found in or between subgroups.

A specific rate is one whose numerator and denominator refer to the same defined category, which represents some aspect of a population, such as age, gender, or place of residence. This rate is calculated by dividing the number of cases in the specific cate-gory (e.g., males between the ages of 15 and 25 years who are sick) by the total population in that same specific category (e.g., the total population of 15- to 25-year-old males).

Adjustments or standardizations of category-specific rates involve a procedure for overall comparison of two or more populations in which background or baseline differences in the distribution of values for a variable (e.g., underlying differences in age) are removed. The procedure is analytical and includes mathematical calculations and transformations for obtaining a summary measure for a population by applying standard weights to the measures within subgroups of the population.

Rate adjustments are often done to identify confounding variables. A *confounding variable* has a direct relationship with two other variables and in some way alters the relationship between those two other variables. To detect a confounding variable, a comparison is made between the association shown by crude data and the association shown after controlling for the suspected confounder. One way is to compare crude data with stratified or specific data (i.e., data depicting values for specific categories). Another way is to determine whether the crude and adjusted measures yield the same conclusions.

Direct adjustment of rates is a useful technique for detecting and controlling confounding effects. Direct adjustment involves the calculation of estimated or expected rates based on a standard population composition. The ratio of adjusted rates provides a measure of the strength of the association when the confounding variable is controlled. If this ratio differs from the ratio of crude rates, then confounding has occurred. The adjusted rate is a weighted mean of the specific rates in the study population using the sizes of the specific groups in the standard population as weights. Direct adjustment can simultaneously control for more than one confounding variable. For instance, to control for both age and gender, age- and gender-specific rates in the study population would be needed, as would the size of the various age and gender categories in the standard population.

The comparison of adjusted rates is not as fully informative, however, as the comparison of specific rates. Adjusted rates can indicate that, when age is controlled, the overall rate for one group may be higher than that of the other group; it cannot, however, tell whether this difference occurs in different age groups. It is advantageous, therefore, to examine specific rates if they are available.

An example of the need for age adjustment of rates is the mortality rates for all causes of death in the United States by age and by race. For both white people and black people, mortality rates begin at high levels during the first years of life, fall to low levels during childhood through young adulthood, and then rise rapidly with increasing age. At every age, however, the death rate for black people exceeds that of white people.[1]

These differences would not be apparent from looking at crude death rates, however. The crude death rate for black people in 1988 was 874 deaths per 100,000 person-years, which is comparable to the corresponding crude death rate for white people, which was 905 deaths per 100,000 person-years. The black-to-white ratio of mortality rates is 0.97, indicating no difference between the races in the rates of death.

Differences in the underlying age distributions of black people and white people explain the errors in this conclusion. On average, black people in the United States are younger than white people. For example, in 1988, only about 9% of black people in the United States were 65 years or older, compared with almost 14% of white people in this age group. Therefore, a smaller proportion of the black population experiences the higher mortality associated with advanced age. In short, to obtain an undistorted summary comparison of mortality for blacks and whites, the age differences between the races must be considered. The usual approach involves removing the influence of age from the comparison of summary rates. This mathematical procedure is known as *direct age-adjustment*.

To calculate an age-adjusted rate, a standard age structure should be selected. By convention, a standard distribution used for age adjustment of mortality rates in the United States is the age distribution of the country's total population in a given year. Next, the age-specific mortality rates for each group being compared is multiplied by the corresponding age-specific number of people in the standard population. The result is the expected number of deaths for that age group. Then the expected number of deaths within each age group is summed to yield the total number of expected deaths for each group being compared (in this case, blacks and whites). Finally, the total number of expected deaths in each group is divided by the total size of the standard population to provide the summary age-adjusted mortality rate.

The numerical values of the age-adjusted rates are not particularly meaningful in and of themselves because the values vary according to the standard age distribution used in the calculation. The utility of age-adjusted rates is that they allow comparison across groups, such as the ratio of black to white mortality rates. In the previous example, the age-adjusted mortality rate for black people was calculated at 789 deaths per 100,000 person-years, whereas the age-adjusted mortality rate for white people was 510 deaths per 100,000 person-years. The black-to-white ratio of mortality rates, once adjusted for the age differences, became 1.55. After the age differences between black people and white people were considered, it was determined that the mortality rate for black people was more than 50 percent greater than it was for white people.

Classification of Disease States

When people begin to exhibit symptoms of, or have, a defined condition, health professionals become concerned about the extent and nature of the disease. For public health officials, the question is always whether further investigation, beyond individual cases, is warranted. Public health investigations take place when—

- The number of people affected with the condition is large, or small but growing quickly
- There are unusual or severe symptoms of a condition
- An obvious explanation for the symptoms or condition is lacking
- There is a need to implement controls, given the extent of the illness
- There is a certain level of public concern about the health problem
- The results of the investigation would contribute to medical knowledge

Diseases are classified in a variety of ways, although typically according to a specific set of symptoms, signs, or other indicators of pathology. *Classification* schemes may be based on the three components of the host–agent–environment model. As such, diseases may be classified by etiological factor, environmental factor, mode of transmission, source or reservoir, or any of its clinical features. Diseases are classified as acute or chronic and can include deficiencies and disabilities as well as communicable and noncommunicable conditions.

In general, there are five major classifications of diseases: (1) congenital and hereditary diseases, (2) allergies and inflammatory diseases, (3) degenerative or chronic diseases, (4) metabolic diseases, and (5) cancer and infectious diseases.[2] Classification of disease or illness is made according to the following categories: allergy, chemical, congenital, hereditary, idiopathic, infectious, inflammatory, metabolic, nutritional, physical agents, psychological, traumatic, and tumors.

Diseases, symptoms, and adverse drug reactions can be misclassified, often leading to misinterpretation of the relationships between exposures or risk factors and symptoms of disease. There are two types of *misclassification*. Nondifferential misclassification is the incorrect categorization of the status of subjects with regard to one variable (exposure) that is unrelated to another characteristic of interest (e.g., disease status). Differential misclassification, in contrast, is the incorrect categorization of the status of subjects with regard to one variable (exposure) that influences other characteristics of interest (e.g., disease status).

For example, adverse reactions to the use of tryptophan were reported in a number of patients in late 1989.[3] Table 2-1 lists the various symptoms reported by affected patients, clinical findings based on examinations, and laboratory values for those patients. A great variety of symptoms, clinical findings, and laboratory values were reported, but not all of the individuals affected with some of these symptoms may be relevant to any study of the cause of these symptoms. Most of the major symptoms, clinical findings, and laboratory values that seem pertinent to the condition defined as an adverse drug reaction syndrome are presented in Table 2-1. In further analysis of this adverse drug reaction outbreak, cases were

TABLE 2-1. **Classification and Misclassification of Adverse Drug Reaction Related to Clinical Features of Eosinophilia-Myalgia Syndrome**

Symptoms	Clinical Findings	Laboratory Values
Muscle pain	*Myalgia*	*Eosinophilia*
Weakness	Increased heart rate	Leukocytosis
Headache	Rash	Elevated serum aldolase
Joint pain	Hepatomegaly	Elevated liver function
Fever	Heart murmur	Elevated erythrocyte
Paresthesias	Swollen eyes	Sedimentation rate
Shortness of breath	Rales	Abnormal chest x-ray
Itching	Abdominal tenderness	Elevated IgE level
Stuffy nose	Edema	
Rapid heartbeat	Bronchospasms	
Nausea	Decreased strength	
Chills	Ascites	
Dry mouth	Decreased sensation	
Cough	Swollen joints	
Extremity swelling		
Rash		
Abdominal pain		
Fatigue		
Malaise		
Swollen eyes		
Vomiting		

Note: Percent of cases experiencing features out of a total number defined as having the syndrome. Features experienced by the greatest percentage of cases are at the top of each list. Features set in italics were used to define the adverse drug reaction outbreak.

TABLE 2-2. **Impact of Nondifferential and Differential Misclassification on Results**

Exposure		Reality EMS Present		Study EMS Present	
		Yes	No	Yes	No
		Nondifferential misclassification			
Tryptophan use	Yes	88	22	54	13
	No	12	78	46	87
		Differential misclassification			
Tryptophan use	Yes	88	22	54	22
	No	12	78	46	78

Note: EMS 5 Eosinophilia-myalgia syndrome.

defined by only one symptom, clinical finding, and laboratory value—those set in italics at the top of each column in the table.

What if the cases had been defined differently, with a greater listing of symptoms, clinical findings, and laboratory values as criteria for determining a case? In trying to assess the relationship between tryptophan use and this syndrome, some subjects—cases and controls—may have made an error when indicating whether they had ever used tryptophan. In reality (as shown in Table 2-2), there is a strong relationship between tryptophan use and the clinical syndrome. The odds ratio, a measure of risk used in case-control studies, is calculated to be 26. In this example, the odds ratio quantifies the probability of developing the syndrome in tryptophan users as compared to nonusers. The OR is discussed in detail in Chapter 6, but can be calculated as follows:

$$OR = \frac{88 \times 78}{22 \times 12} = 26$$

There was a 26 times greater risk of developing the syndrome in individuals who had used tryptophan compared with those who had not used it.

In the example of nondifferential misclassification, 39% of the cases (individuals with the syndrome) misidentified their use of tryptophan and, thus, a smaller number of them were labeled as having used tryptophan (and a greater number were labeled as nonusers when compared to reality). For the control group, 41% mislabeled their tryptophan use. A lesser number than in reality reported using tryptophan than had actually done so. As a result, the odds ratio was calculated as 7.9, still a very high degree of risk, indicating a strong relationship between tryptophan use and the syndrome.

$$OR = \frac{54 \times 87}{46 \times 13} = \frac{4698}{598} = 7.9$$

The misclassification of tryptophan use occurred in both cases and controls, so the relative impact on assessing the true relationship between use and the syndrome was not great.

In the second example, of differential misclassification, only individuals with the syndrome misidentified their use of tryptophan. In fact, 39% of the cases mislabeled their tryptophan use as nonuse. As a result, a smaller number of cases was classified as tryptophan users, whereas the control subjects who were tryptophan users were correctly labeled and counted. The odds ratio was calculated as 4.2, compared with the original measure of risk of 26.

$$OR = \frac{54 \times 78}{46 \times 22} = \frac{4212}{1012} = 4.2$$

Although a 4 times greater risk is significant, the strength of the relationship was greatly reduced due to misclassification of tryptophan use by some cases.

Outbreaks or Epidemics of Disease

Health problems typically are first viewed when individual patients report to a health care facility. A few patients with a specific health problem may not increase alertness about larger-scale problems in the whole population. If there is a hint of a larger problem, usually indicated by a greatly increasing number of people with the same problem, then epidemiological investigation may become warranted.

A classic example of this process occurs with a food-borne *outbreak* or *epidemic*. A few individuals present at a health facility or see a professional with a set of specific symptoms. If a larger problem is suspected or if more people could develop the disease for the same reason the first few were infected, then a response to protect the health of the general public becomes necessary. The patients involved in the outbreak and those who are not exhibiting symptoms but may have been exposed are studied. All types of data are collected from these subjects (sick and well), including personal data (e.g., demographics, behaviors, exposures, symptoms), clinical data (e.g., clinical examination findings, laboratory results), and environmental data (e.g., description of setting; chemical and biological data; interpersonal and social data; data on causative agents, exposures, risk factors, or potential sources of the problem).

The overall natural history of a specific disease can be determined with the use of these data. For an outbreak, or an epidemic, an epidemic curve can be constructed to determine the onset times, first cases and total number of people involved, incubation period, and duration of the epidemic.

Incubation period: interval of time between exposure to (contact with) causative agent (risk factor) and onset of the condition (symptoms, disease).

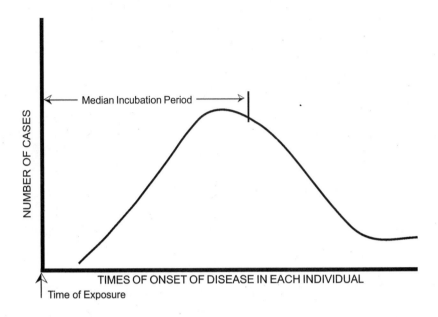

Figure 2-3. Example of an epidemic curve. (Adapted from Ref. 2.)

The incubation period is determined from the epidemic curve. The median incubation period is the median point on the curve; by this point, 50% of the cases have occurred in a single-source, common-vehicle outbreak. As can be seen in Figure 2-3, the distribution of individual times of onset for specific diseases is plotted to create an epidemic curve. This curve represents all of the individual patient incubation periods for the outbreak.

Assessing the Source, Nature, and Extent of a Specific Outbreak

Many aspects of the nature and extent of an outbreak can be determined from the data collected from individuals who are involved or thought to be exposed. The source of the problem, its mode of transmission and incubation period, and the affected people in a population can be determined through analysis of the data and information collected from the subjects. It is important to remember that, for an account or description of an outbreak to be descriptive, it must be seen in proportion to the rest of the group or population in which it occurs. The following measures are important in assessing an outbreak or an epidemic.

Attack rate (AR): proportion of people in a population who develop a particular condition during an outbreak (specified time period); also called *crude attack rate.*

$$AR = \frac{\text{number of new cases (number with disease)}}{\text{number of people at risk (exposed to contagion)}} \text{ per unit of time}$$

Food-specific attack rate: proportion of people in a population who develop a condition after eating a specific food. An attack rate is calculated both for the people who ate a specific food item and for those who did not eat the specific food item.

AR (for those who ate item)

$$= \frac{\text{number of people who ate specific food and became sick}}{\text{total number of people who ate specific food}}$$

AR (for those who did not eat item)

$$= \frac{\text{number of people who did } not \text{ eat specific food and became sick}}{\text{total number of people who did } not \text{ eat specific food}}$$

These rates are compared to determine the source of the food-borne disease (often by calculating a ratio of attack rates, called a *risk ratio*). The two attack rates can then be compared to determine the likelihood that eating the food was associated with becoming sick. Risk estimates can be used to quantify such associations. They will be discussed in detail in Chapter 6

Case Study: Outbreak of Food Poisoning in New Dorm Cafeteria

This case study is an example of a food-borne, infectious disease outbreak. The measures and calculations used here assess the source, nature, and spread of the outbreak.

During the winter break after the holidays, a number of students who had been living in the new dorm returned the week before school resumed. The new dorm's cafeteria had been serving them 2 meals a day, breakfast and dinner. On late Wednesday morning, students began to appear at the school nurse's office reporting symptoms of nausea, vomiting, dizziness, and fever. The dean of students wants to know what is going on. She asks you to determine the source of this disease outbreak.

Forty-five students were living in the new dorm on the day of the outbreak. You locate and interview all 45 of them, thereby collecting the data presented in Table 2-3. To prepare a report for the dean, you need to complete the following steps:

1. Describe the demographic makeup of the students who became ill and those who did not.

2. Construct an epidemic curve, and determine the time of onset and incubation period for this outbreak.

3. Calculate attack rates for each food item served by the cafeteria that morning, and identify the probable source of the outbreak.

4. Determine the prevalence for this disease in the dorm student population by late afternoon that day. What was the incidence rate for the 1-hour period, 11:45 A.M. to 12:45 P.M. (inclusive)?

5. Comment on how the new cafeteria might prevent another such outbreak in the future.

Analyzing Characteristics of the Outbreak

The first step in analyzing this disease outbreak is to focus on the number of people affected and whether any specific variables (demographic variables, such as gender and year in school) seem to indicate a relationship to the disase. The demographic makeup of the students who became sick is as follows:

$$AR = 35 \text{ students became ill}/45 \text{ students living in the dorm}$$

$$AR = \frac{35}{45} \times 100 = 78\%$$

More than three quarters of the new dorm's residents became ill (i.e., contracted the disease) during this outbreak, which lasted for less than 24 hours. Calculation of gender-specific attack rates and attack rates for students in different school years are as follows:

$$AR \text{ (females)} = \frac{18}{20} \times 100 = 90\%$$

$$AR \text{ (males)} = \frac{17}{25} \times 100 = 68\%$$

$$\text{Risk ratio (females to males)} = \frac{90}{68} = 1.3$$

Female students living in the dorm were at 1.3 times greater risk than male students for contracting this disease during the outbreak, a slightly greater but not significant risk.

$$AR \text{ (freshmen)} = \frac{25}{31} \times 100 = 81\%$$

$$AR \text{ (sophomores)} = \frac{9}{13} \times 100 = 69\%$$

$$AR \text{ (juniors)} = \frac{1}{1} \times 100 = 100\%$$

TABLE 2-3. Raw Data from Disease Outbreak in New Dorm Cafeteria

Student	Sex	Year	Time at Breakfast	Time at Nurse	Ham	Sausage	Oatmeal	Eggs	French Toast	Pancakes	Muffins
1	M	F	7:30 A.M.	10:30 A.M.	Y	N	N	Y	N	Y	Y
2	F	S	8:45 A.M.	11:15 A.M.	N	Y	N	Y	Y	N	Y
3	F	F	8:00 A.M.	11:00 A.M.	N	N	Y	N	N	Y	Y
4	M	F	8:15 A.M.	9:15 A.M.	Y	N	N	Y	Y	N	N
5	M	S	7:45 A.M.	11:45 A.M.	N	Y	N	Y	N	Y	Y
6	M	S	8:45 A.M.	not sick	Y	N	Y	N	N	Y	N
7	M	F	9:00 A.M.	12:30 P.M.	Y	Y	N	Y	N	Y	Y
8	F	F	8:00 A.M.	12:30 P.M.	N	Y	N	Y	Y	Y	Y
9	M	S	8:30 A.M.	not sick	N	Y	N	N	N	N	N
10	F	F	8:15 A.M.	11:45 A.M.	N	N	Y	Y	N	N	Y
11	F	F	7:45 A.M.	10:15 A.M.	N	N	N	Y	N	Y	Y
12	M	F	8:30 A.M.	10:30 A.M.	Y	Y	N	N	Y	N	Y
13	M	F	9:00 A.M.	not sick	Y	Y	Y	Y	N	Y	Y
14	M	F	8:00 A.M.	11:00 A.M.	N	Y	N	N	N	Y	Y
15	F	S	8:15 A.M.	11:45 A.M.	Y	Y	Y	Y	Y	Y	Y
16	F	J	9:00 A.M.	11:30 A.M.	N	Y	N	N	N	N	Y
17	M	F	8:45 A.M.	not sick	N	N	Y	N	N	N	Y
18	M	S	7:45 A.M.	9:45 A.M.	Y	N	N	Y	N	N	N
19	F	F	8:30 A.M.	10:00 A.M.	N	N	Y	Y	N	Y	Y
20	M	F	8:30 A.M.	11:30 A.M.	N	Y	N	Y	Y	Y	N
21	F	S	8:30 A.M.	12:30 P.M.	Y	N	Y	Y	Y	Y	Y
22	M	F	8:15 A.M.	not sick	N	Y	N	N	Y	N	N
23	M	F	9:00 A.M.	1:30 P.M.	N	Y	N	N	Y	N	Y

#	Sex	Year	Time at breakfast	Time at nurse							
24	F	F	8:15 A.M.	10:45 A.M.	N	Y	Y	Y	Y	Y	N
25	M	F	9:00 A.M.	2:30 P.M.	Y	N	N	N	Y	Y	Y
26	F	S	8:30 A.M.	not sick	Y	Y	N	N	Y	N	Y
27	F	F	8:30 A.M.	not sick	Y	N	N	N	Y	N	Y
28	F	F	8:30 A.M.	1:30 P.M.	N	Y	Y	Y	N	N	N
29	M	F	8:45 A.M.	2:45 P.M.	N	N	N	N	N	N	Y
30	F	F	8:30 A.M.	12:30 P.M.	N	Y	N	Y	N	Y	Y
31	M	F	9:00 A.M.	12:30 P.M.	Y	Y	N	Y	N	N	Y
32	F	F	8:00 A.M.	10:30 A.M.	N	N	N	Y	Y	N	Y
33	M	F	7:45 A.M.	10:45 A.M.	N	Y	Y	Y	N	N	Y
34	M	F	8:00 A.M.	not sick	Y	N	Y	N	Y	Y	Y
35	M	S	9:00 A.M.	12:30 P.M.	N	N	Y	N	N	N	Y
36	M	S	8:30 A.M.	11:00 A.M.	N	Y	N	Y	Y	N	Y
37	M	S	7:45 A.M.	not sick	Y	Y	N	Y	N	Y	N
38	F	F	8:30 A.M.	12:00 P.M.	N	N	N	N	Y	N	Y
39	M	S	8:30 A.M.	11:00 A.M.	Y	Y	Y	Y	N	N	Y
40	F	F	8:30 A.M.	12:00 P.M.	Y	Y	N	Y	Y	N	N
41	M	F	8:15 A.M.	not sick	N	N	Y	N	N	N	Y
42	F	F	8:15 A.M.	12:15 P.M.	Y	Y	N	Y	N	Y	N
43	F	F	8:00 A.M.	11:30 A.M.	N	N	Y	N	N	Y	Y
44	M	F	7:45 A.M.	10:45 A.M.	Y	Y	N	Y	Y	Y	N
45	F	S	8:00 A.M.	11:00 A.M.	Y	N	N	Y	Y	N	Y

Note: Sex: F = Female, M = Male.
Year: F = Freshman, S = Sophomore, J = Junior.
Time at breakfast: Time student began eating.
Time at nurse: Time student reported to school nurse.
Y: Yes (eaten).
N: No (not eaten).

There is little difference in attack rates among students from the first 3 years in school.

Constructing an Epidemic Curve

The epidemic curve for this outbreak is constructed by plotting the individual incubation periods. Using the data in Table 2-3, individual incubation periods can be calculated for the individuals who reported sick to the school nurse by subtracting the time when they ate breakfast from the time when they first reported to the nurse (e.g., student #1 reported to the nurse at 10:30 A.M. and had eaten breakfast at 7:30 A.M.; incubation period = 10:30 − 7:30 = 3-hour incubation period for student #1). Taking the individual incubation periods for each sick student and plotting them by the number of cases exhibiting the same incubation time results in the epidemic curve for this outbreak (Figure 2-4).

The onset of the disease outbreak was within 1 hour of exposure, eating breakfast (first case, 1 person within 1 hour after eating). The incubation period for this disease outbreak is 3 hours. This was determined by locating the median, or middle, case in the total group of sick people. This curve represents 35 sick people so the middle case (point in time at which 50% of the cases have occurred) is technically the time-point for case #17.5. By convention, when there is an odd number of cases, the median case can be the one before or after the half-fraction (0.5). In this example, either case #17 or case #18 can represent the median case (both of which occur in the 3.0 hour time period, as the cases are counted from the earliest to the latest incubation times.

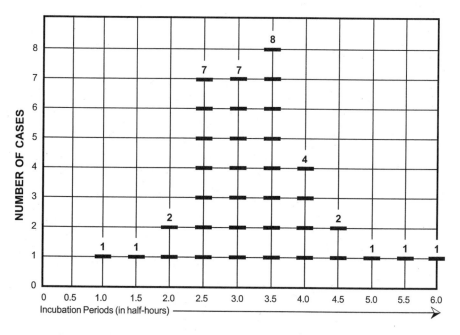

Figure 2-4. Epidemic curve for food-borne outbreak.

Identifying the Source of the Outbreak

The attack rates for individual food items served by the cafeteria during break-fast are compiled in Table 2-4. The risk ratio for the subjects who ate a specific food item compared with those who did not eat it is calculated by dividing the attack rate for those who ate the food by the attack rate for those who did not eat it. Risks ratios for the food items range from 0.91 to 1.05—basically, no difference in risk between those who ate each item and those who did not—with one exception. For those who ate the eggs, the risk of developing gastroenteritis was 1.5 times greater than for those who did not eat them (Risk Ratio = 92%/60% = 1.53). In short, the source of this outbreak was the eggs.

Prevalence and Incidence of Gastroenteritis

By the end of the outbreak, the prevalence was the same number as the overall attack rate, 78% (P = number of existing cases/number in population = 35/45 × 100 = 78%).

The incidence for the 1-hour period of 11:45 A.M. to 12:45 P.M. was calculated to determine the outbreak's rate of growth. Incidence is calculated with the number of new cases divided by the number of people in the population still at risk. (Remember that a number of the students in this population had already reported to the school nurse by 11:45 A.M. and, thus, were no longer at risk.)

$$\mathbf{IR} \, (11\text{:}45 \, \text{A.M.}\text{--}12\text{:}45 \, \text{P.M.}) = \frac{12 \text{ new cases}}{45 - 19} = \frac{12}{26} \times 100 = 46\%$$

TABLE 2-4. **Attack Rates for Food Items By Subjects Who Ate and Those Who Did Not**

Food Item	Ate Food Item				Did Not Eat Food Item				Risk Ratio
	Sick	Not Sick	Total	Attack Rate (%)	Sick	Not Sick	Total	Attack Rate (%)	
Ham	14	5	19	74	21	5	26	81	0.91
Sausage	19	5	24	79	16	5	21	76	1.04
Oatmeal	12	4	16	75	23	6	29	79	0.95
Eggs	23	2	25	92	12	8	20	60	1.53
French toast	16	4	20	80	19	6	25	76	1.05
Pancakes	17	5	22	77	18	5	23	78	0.99
Muffins	24	7	31	77	11	3	14	79	0.97

Public Health Prevention of Outbreaks

This food-borne gastroenteritis outbreak was caused by an infectious agent in contaminated food served by the cafeteria at breakfast. To prevent future outbreaks or occurrences of this disease, good sanitary food-handling and storage practices must be employed. These practices would include employee cleanliness (e.g., washing hands before food preparation), prohibiting sick employees from handling food, cleaner facilities and equipment, better refrigeration of prepared foods, and preparing food items closer to their serving times (instead of storing them).

Secondary Attack Rate

Secondary attack rates are used in infectious disease investigations when a limited timeframe exists and the infectious agent has a short incubation period. Secondary attack rates are often used for cases of illness that occur in the same household or work group, when the primary case of disease is present. The relevant timeframe is before other people in the group contract the disease. When other people in the group come down with a disease that was transmitted by the primary group with the infection, they are considered to be secondary cases.

The risk of coming down with a condition for the secondary cases is an aspect of the *secondary attack rate*. The number of people who had contact with, or were exposed to, the primary source of the infection within the infectious agent's incubation period is used to calculate the rate. The numerator in the secondary attack rate includes the number of cases of disease that occurred within the same group or household following the onset of the primary, or first, case and those who are infected by that primary case. The denominator excludes individuals who had immunizations or currently or previously had the disease and are now immune.

Secondary attack rate (Sec. AR): a measure of the degree of a spread of a disease within a group that has been exposed to a causative agent by contact with a case.

$$\text{Sec. AR} = \frac{\text{number of exposed people developing disease within incubation period (specified time)}}{\text{total number of people exposed to primary case}}$$

Summary

In this chapter, the concept of medical surveillance was introduced. This approach of monitoring data to determine changes in the health status of a population is also used to determine patterns of drug use and the occurrence of drug use problems in a population. The concept of epidemic, or disease outbreak, was also introduced as the foundation for many epidemiological investigations of problems in health care and drug use.

References

1. National Center for Health Statistics. Advance report of final mortality statistics, 1988. *Monthly Vital Stat* 1990; 39 (Suppl).

2. Lilienfeld DE, Stolley PD. *Foundations of Epidemiology*. 3rd ed. New York, NY: Oxford University Press; 1994.

3. Centers for Disease Control and Prevention. Update: Eosinophilia-myalgia syndrome associated with ingestion of L-tryptophan—United States as of January 9, 1990. *MMWR Morb Mortal Wkly Rep* 1990; 39: 14–15.

Study Questions

1. The ratio of male-to-female age-adjusted mortality rates in the United States for pneumonia and influenza is 1.7. This means that compared to the age-adjusted mortality rate for females, the rate for males is—

    a. 7% higher

    b. 17% higher

    c. 70% higher

    d. 17% lower

    e. 70% lower

2. The interval of time between exposure to a causative agent or a risk factor and the onset of symptoms or a disease is called—

    a. epidemic outbreak

    b. attack rate

    c. incubation period

    d. infectious period

3. The proportion of people who have a particular condition and who die from it in a given time period is called—

    a. survival rate

    b. secondary attack rate

    c. mortality rate

    d. case fatality rate

4. Define the following terms:

    a. medical surveillance

    b. proportion

    c. rate

    d. morbidity

    e. mortality

    f. prevalence

    g. period prevalence

h. incidence rate

i. cumulative incidence

j. incidence rate in person-time units

k. survival rate

l. rate adjustment

m. classification

n. misclassification

o. outbreak or epidemic

p. attack rate

q. food-specific attack rate

r. secondary attack rate

5. If a person is exposed to a contagion, causative agent, or risk factor, he or she will eventually develop the condition or disease.

a. True

b. False

6. In a case-control study of maternal cigarette smoking as a hazard for low birth weight, it appeared that the mothers of children with low birth weight underreported the extent of their cigarette smoking compared with the mothers of normal birth weight babies.

a) This is an example of—

a. confounding

b. validity but not reliability

c. misclassification

d. nonrandom sampling

b) As a result of this problem, the risk that was calculated was probably—

a. inflated (too high)

b. deflated (too low)

c. unchanged

d. changed, but the direction cannot be known

7. What is the relationship among point prevalence, period prevalence, and incidence?

8. What factors can affect the prevalence of a disease in a population?

9. In calculating an incidence rate, what part of the population is included in the denominator?

10. In a small town with an adult population of 1275, an initial clinical examina-

tion reveals that 117 individuals have diabetes mellitus. During the following 10 years, 59 additional people develop diabetes.

a. What is the initial prevalence of diabetes in this town?

b. What is the risk (10-year incidence) of developing diabetes in this small town?

11. In a postmarketing surveillance study, you wish to assess the risk of *Candida vaginitis* to users of your new oral contraceptive (OC) product. In a large health maintenance organization population, you identify 2194 users of your new OC and 12,161 nonusers. During 1998, there were 28 new cases of *Candida vaginitis* in the user population and 53 cases of *Candida vaginitis* in the nonuser population. Calculate the incidence rate (per 1000) in each group and compare the risk of developing vaginitis if a patient was taking the new OC product.

12. During an 8-hour work shift at the new Registry of Motor Vehicles building, 30 employees (20 females and 10 males) developed the following symptoms: nausea, vomiting, headaches, and dizziness. These affected individuals went to their family doctors, were treated, and were released. In an attempt to describe this outbreak of symptoms, you are asked to assess the situation and to perform some calculations.

a. Six hundred people worked in the building. What was the attack rate?

b. Of those 600 employees, 350 were females and 250 were males. Calculate which gender, if either, was at greater risk for coming down with the symptoms.

c. All 570 of the remaining employees were surveyed to see if other people had experienced these symptoms. Four hundred survey forms were returned. Eighty employees reported symptoms consistent with the syndrome observed in the workers who sought medical attention. Based on these survey data, what was the attack rate?

d. Would you report the attack rate based on those who went to their doctor or based on the survey data? Explain your answer.

Chapter 3

Observational Study Designs

One of two major approaches in conducting epidemiological investigations involves observation of the disease, drug use problem, or other phenomenon of interest. The other major approach, called *experimental epidemiology,* is discussed in Chapter 4.

Study designs used in observational epidemiology include case reports, cross-sectional studies, case-control studies, and cohort studies. Studies can be designed to be retrospective or prospective. In all of these study designs, sampling, or how people are or are not chosen to be studied, is an important issue. It is a primary way to differentiate among designs. In this chapter, each of the major observational study designs is described, and the process for conducting them is outlined.

Observational study designs in pharmacoepidemiology produce data and information that identify the occurrence of drug use problems and that test hypotheses regarding the probable reasons or causes of these problems. In some instances, instead of a problem resulting from drug use, new beneficial uses for a drug product might be identified for further investigation in clinical trials.

Each epidemiological investigation follows the same general rules of research design and methodology. First, the problem must be identified or the research question must be stated. Dependent variable(s), the outcome(s), and the independent variable(s) are identified. The causes or things associated with the disease or drug use problem are the independent variables. Second, cases are defined, or populations at risk are sampled. Other steps in the process include identifying and collecting all of the relevant data and information, analyzing the data according to the study hypotheses or research questions, and interpreting the results. Analysis may include subdividing the population according to a certain risk factor and comparing rates for each subgroup.

Observational Epidemiology

Epidemiological study designs also can be described according to a number of different aspects. One aspect is whether the study is observational or experimental. Investigators in observational studies may plan and identify variables to be measured, but human intervention is not a part of the process. Experimental studies, in contrast, involve intervention in ongoing processes to study any resulting change or difference. Epidemiological studies are also descriptive or analytical in nature. Descriptive studies attempt to uncover and portray the occurrence of the condition or problem, whereas analytical studies determine the causes of the condition or problem.

Observational epidemiology provides information about disease patterns or drug use problems by various characteristics of person, place, and time. This approach is used by public health professionals for efficient allocation of resources and to target populations for education, prevention, and treatment programs. It also is used by epidemiologists to generate hypotheses regarding the causes of disease or drug use problems. Some researchers do not consider experimental studies to be true epidemiological studies in the traditional sense because they follow clinical or planned research designs. Descriptive studies provide insight, data, and information about the course or patterns of disease or drug use problems in a population or group. Analytical studies are used to test cause–effect relationships, and they usually rely on the generation of new data.

There are five general types of epidemiological study design: (1) case reports and case series, (2) cross-sectional studies, (3) case-control studies, (4) cohort studies, and (5) experiments. A *case report* is a descriptive study of a single patient, and a *case series* is a collection of case reports. A *cross-sectional study* is a prevalence study—a basic descriptive study that examines relationships between a disease or drug use problem and other characteristics of people in a population at one point in time. A case-control study compares people who have the disease or problem (cases) to those who do not (controls) with respect to characteristics of interest (i.e., potential causes). A *cohort study* is an incidence study that measures characteristics or attributes in a population free of a disease or drug use problem and relates them to subsequent development of the disease in that population as it is followed over time. This type of study is also referred to as a *longitudinal study.* *Experimental studies* are clinical trials and intervention studies designed to compare outcomes between two or more treatment or intervention groups.

These different aspects and relationships of epidemiological study designs are summarized and portrayed in Figure 3-1.[1] At the basic level, investigators can exert control over the process by assigning subjects to study groups, such as in experiments, or they do not exert control and only observe what is occurring naturally. Experimental studies are further divided into studies that assess effects or outcomes in individual subjects or studies that assess effects in communities or large groups of people. Observational studies are divided into descriptive or analytical types, with the latter type being further defined by the focus of sampling for the exposure or disease.

Retrospective and Prospective Designs

Epidemiological studies also can be either retrospective or prospective. In a retrospective design, the research question or hypothesis is conceived and studied using data that were collected and recorded previously (before the design of the current study). In a prospective, or longitudinal, design, the collection of data is planned in

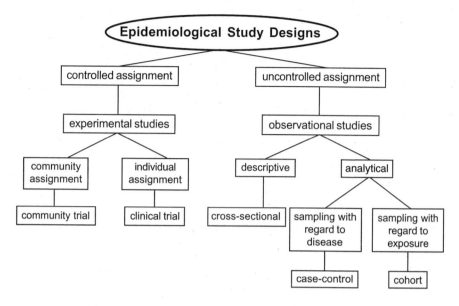

Figure 3-1. Aspects and relationships of epidemiological methods. (Adapted from Ref. 1.)

advance and actually occurs after the study has begun. The advantages and disadvantages of retrospective versus prospective study designs are summarized in Table 3-1.

Exposure, Disease, and Data Collection in Study Designs

The temporal relationships among exposure and identification, disease identification, and data collection in each of the epidemiological study designs are illustrated in Figure 3-2. Epidemiological investigations focus on identifying people (cases) with diseases or drug use problems, identifying the exposure (e.g., causative agent, risk factor) associated with the development of that disease or problem, and determining when the exposure occurred. As discussed, the other key difference between study designs involves when the data are collected and recorded. [2,3]

Case reports are not illustrated in Figure 3-2 because they simply involve the collection of data on one subject when the event occurs. In a cross-sectional study, data collection occurs only once (not over an extended period); thus, the inquiry is only at one point in time. The length of the study is usually the time it takes to collect, record, and analyze the data. As the data are analyzed, subjects with certain diseases (cases) and exposures are identified. Obviously, exposures and outcomes must have occurred before the study was initiated and the data were collected.

In a case-control study, data have been collected and recorded before the study was initiated. The direction of inquiry is back in time, and exposures have occurred beforehand. As in a cross-sectional study, both exposure and disease (cases) are identified through data analysis. In a case-control study, however, data

TABLE 3-1. **Comparison of Retrospective and Prospective Approaches**

Retrospective	Prospective
Inexpensive to conduct	Expensive to conduct
Completed in a shorter time period	Completed over a longer time period
Easier to access a larger number of subjects	More difficult to access subjects and usually requires a larger number of subjects
Allows results to be obtained more quickly	Exposure status and diagnostic methods for disease may change
Useful for studying exposures that no longer occur	Loss of subjects from the study over time may be substantial
Information and data may be less complete and inaccurate	Information and data may be more complete and accurate
Subjects may not remember past information	Direct access to study subjects enhances reliability of data

were collected beforehand, and they are assembled and analyzed with the present study's objectives in mind.

Cohort studies involve following a group of subjects, who were free of the outcome of interest (e.g., disease, drug use problem) at the beginning of the study, over an extended period. The direction of inquiry is most commonly forward in time. To determine that all study subjects are initially free of the disease, cohort studies often begin with a cross-sectional study. Potential subjects determined to have the disease would then be excluded from the cohort study. Data collection and recording continue to occur (multiple times) throughout the length of the cohort study. As subjects are monitored over time, exposure occurrences are identified, as is the subsequent development of disease.

In a clinical trial, the notions of exposure and disease identification are reoriented to the nature of trial design. The direction of inquiry is forward in time. Clinical and community intervention trials are experiments in which a proportion of subjects are given a new treatment or intervention; essentially, they are exposed to a beneficial agent, such as a new drug. The remaining subjects do not receive the experimental treatment. Data are collected and recorded for the length of the study, and the beneficial result or outcome is measured to determine if the new treatment was successful. The design of a clinical trial is similar to that of a cohort study, but a clinical trial involves active human intervention, whereas a cohort study passively observes a naturally occurring process.

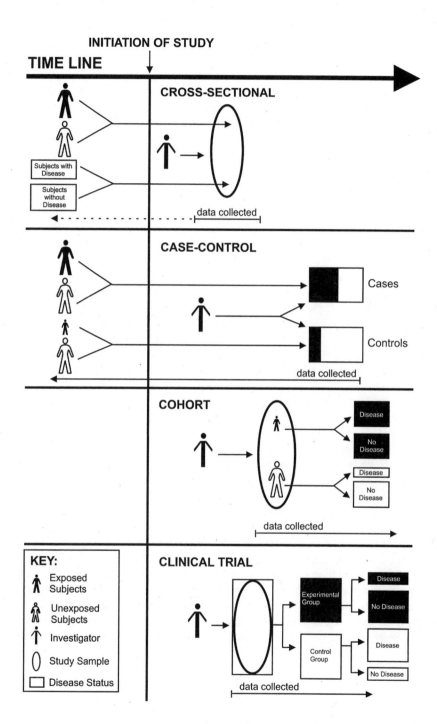

Figure 3-2. Epidemiological study designs.

These relationships are traditional, but they are not mutually exclusive to certain study designs. Although cohort studies are traditionally known to be prospective in nature, epidemiologists have designed retrospective cohort studies. Similarly, although the data for case-control studies have typically been collected before the study was initiated, many investigators in these studies have revisited subjects after the study has been initiated and collected new data while the study is in progress to supplement the previously collected data. Future efforts by epidemiologists will result in new "hybrid" study designs that improve on the traditional designs while attending to issues of cost, time, and sample size.

Descriptive Studies

Descriptive studies include case reports, case series, cross-sectional surveys, and analyses of data collected routinely over time through various databases (e.g., medical surveillance). As noted previously, a case report is a descriptive study of one individual, and a case series involves a number of individual case reports that have been collected together. In these situations, an astute clinician finds unusual features of a disease or effects of a drug, or the patient's medical history, that lead to the formulation of a new research question or hypothesis.

Case reports are the most common type of study published in the medical literature. They note unusual medical occurrences, identify new diseases, and describe adverse effects from drug therapies. Clinical investigators can use challenge–rechallenge data to help establish causality. In this approach, administration of a drug (the challenge) might be suspected of producing a specific symptom (side effect or adverse reaction). Administration of the drug can be stopped to observe whether the side effect or adverse reaction diminishes. If it does, then administration of the drug can be resumed (the rechallenge) to observe whether the effect returns, suggesting a possible relationship between the two events. There are no incidence data in case reports or case series. These reports are obviously a very low-cost approach to identifying problems.

A case series is an attempt to quantify the numerator—the number of people with the problem. If the population is known, then a denominator can be selected to calculate a rate. There is, however, no control group for comparison.

Cross-sectional studies (sometimes called *ecological studies*) examine the characteristics of a population. These studies are used to describe disease or drug use problems in relation to some factor of interest. Comparing cigarette consumption with rates of cancer, and alcohol consumption with coronary heart disease mortality, are examples of descriptive studies that first identified strong relationships between disease and behavior. Routine databases also provide information for descriptive studies. Vital statistic records provide information on mortality, and surveillance programs report on morbidity.

There are many problems with descriptive methods. In case reports and case series, there is no control group. For cross-sectional studies, there are confounding factors that might mask the true impact of risk factors. Cross-sectional studies present only a snapshot of the problem, such as disease or drug use, in a population.

Investigators must be cautious when looking at trends over time and across settings. Measured trends may not be caused by actual changes in the occurrence of a disease but, instead, might be due to changes in diagnostic techniques, reporting mechanisms, disease definition, treatment improvements, changes in survival rate, accuracy in population enumeration, or changes in the age distribution of the population. Special caution is also needed in interpreting mortality statistics because mortality is a combination of disease incidence and duration. Although death certificate data are readily available, they can be incomplete and inaccurate.

Sampling

Sampling is the process of identifying and selecting subjects to be study participants. Sampling involves drawing a smaller group of people from a larger population or group. If sufficient attention is not paid to sampling, systematic error can arise in subject selection.

There are five types of sampling. *Nonrandom sampling* simply involves choosing people, perhaps in no particular order or according to no logical structure. An example of nonrandom sampling is the selection of every patient who comes into a clinic on a specific day. *Systematic sampling* involves selecting a fraction or part (percentage) of the population under study based on a particular order or listing of the members of the population. For instance, if 10% of the population is selected to be the sample, then a listing of the population is developed, and every 10th person on the list is selected to be a part of the sample.

Simple random sampling involves a process in which each person has an equal chance of being selected directly from the population. *Stratified random sampling* involves the process of dividing the population into strata, or subgroups, according to a specific variable or characteristic and randomly sampling or selecting from the subgroups. The sample collected is compared to the population from which it was chosen to see how closely it represents that population. This process can allow for oversampling of specific groups. *Cluster sampling* involves a process of dividing the population into subgroups called *clusters* (not as homogeneous as strata), randomly sampling clusters, and then possibly selecting a random sample of people in each cluster.

Cross-Sectional Study Design

Cross-sectional studies are sometimes called *prevalence studies*. They are studies of total populations or population groups in which information is collected about the present and past characteristics, behaviors, or experiences of individuals.

There are a number of advantages in performing a cross-sectional study. These studies involve a single data collection and, thus, are less expensive and more expedient to conduct. They provide information and data useful for the planning of health services and medical programs. They also provide a one-time glimpse at the study population, showing the relative distribution of conditions, diseases, and injuries—and their attributes—in a group or population. Cross-sectional studies can be of value in predicting the future spread of certain diseases. They are based on a sample of the whole population and do not rely on individuals presenting themselves for medical treatment.

Cross-sectional studies have disadvantages, too. They cannot show cause–effect relationships. The results are representative only of the individuals who participate in the study, provide accurate information, are surveyed, and are identified as having the disease. This design is not effective if the level of disease rate is very small. Seasonal variations of disease are not well represented in cross-sectional studies, depending on when the study is performed. These studies have limited value in predicting future occurrence of some diseases. They are more effective in identifying chronic diseases and problems and less effective in identifying communicable diseases of short incubation periods and short durations.

Case-Control Study Design

The case-control design is an analytical, retrospective study comparing people with the disease (cases) to a sample of people without the disease (controls) with respect to exposures or characteristics of interest. This type of study is done to identify factors that could be responsible for the development of a disease or drug use problem.

Case control studies have several important advantages. This design provides an efficient means to study disease, and it is more feasible than other types of investigations because fewer subjects are required. Smaller sample size requirements, along with prior data collection, are accompanied by reduced costs. This type of study also allows an investigator to study several risk factors for a single disease, and it can provide or suggest evidence of an association that warrants public health intervention to reduce exposure to the risk factor. It is practical for studying chronic diseases with long latency periods.

The case-control design has disadvantages, too. Cases and controls are not representative of the whole population. There is no direct measure of incidence or prevalence. It is inefficient in situations where exposure is rare. There can be major problems with bias in subject recall, exclusion criteria, determining that the exposure precedes disease, and bias in selection criteria.

Case-control studies are designed to assess association between disease occurrence and exposures (e.g., causative agents, risk factors) suspected of causing or preventing the disease. The case-control study is the primary design for determining associations between drug use and side effects or adverse reactions. In many situations, a case-control study is more efficient than a cohort study because a smaller sample size is required. One key feature of a case-control study, which distinguishes it from a cohort study, is the selection of subjects based on disease status. The investigator selects cases from among people who have the disease of interest and controls from among those who do not. Cases are selected from a clearly defined population called the *source population*. Controls are chosen from the same population yielding the cases. Prior exposure histories of cases and controls are examined to assess relationships between exposure and disease.

The basic steps in a case control study consist of formulation of the research questions; identification and collection of cases; selection of controls and matching; determination of exposure in all subjects; and collection, analysis, and interpretation of the study data.

The first step in a case-control study, beyond the research question, is to identify and select cases, a step that determines the source population. In some situations, complete identification of cases in a well-defined source population may be too time consuming or otherwise impossible.

Selecting Cases and Controls

Identification and collection of cases involves specifying the criteria for defining a person as a case—in other words, as having the disease (also called *case definition*). This definition consists of a set of criteria, also called *eligibility criteria,* for inclusion in the study. There also are criteria for exclusion from the study. Cases are found through registries, health care systems, and other sources that identify new or incidence cases. For example, cases may be sampled from those admitted to particular hospitals or clinics. The most important step in designing a case-control study is to specify the case definition.

It is important to minimize the likelihood that true cases are missed (the criteria must be sensitive) but, at the same time, falsely classifying nondiseased people as cases must be avoided (the criteria must be specific). In practice, study inclusion criteria are chosen to minimize misclassification yet retain feasibility. Other sources of cases can be all cases diagnosed in the community (from, e.g., hospitals, medical facilities, physicians' office); cases diagnosed in a sample of the general population; cases diagnosed in all hospitals in the community; and cases diagnosed in a single hospital.

The next step is selection of the controls. Controls are chosen from the source population. The source population is usually defined by geographic area. It is important to select controls so that participation does not depend on exposure.

The ideal situation is a random sample from the same source population as the cases. Investigators may use more than one control group. Controls can be selected by sampling the general population in the same community; the hospital community (patients in the same hospital); individuals who reside in the same block or neighborhood; and spouses, siblings, or associates (schoolmates, co-workers) of the cases.

Once cases and controls are selected, information must be collected on prior exposure to the risk factor(s) of interest. Information concerning a variety of exposures may be collected to look for associations with the disease or drug use. Interviews and questionnaires are the most common means of determining a subject's exposure history and medical records review is another source, but the most objective means for characterizing exposure is the use of a biological marker.

Matching Cases and Controls

Matching is a popular approach to control for confounding and selection bias in case-control studies. Its popularity reflects the notion that matching cases and controls helps to ensure that these groups are similar with respect to important risk factors, thereby making case-control comparisons less subject to confounding or selection bias. The first step in matching is to identify a case. One or more potential controls, with the same or very similar values for each matching factor as the case, are then selected from the source population. For instance, matching may be made on gender and age group. More than one control can be matched with each case, although the ratio of controls to cases typically does not exceed 4 to 1.

Matching can increase the statistical efficiency of case-control comparisons. It can achieve a specified level of statistical power with a smaller sample size. A matching protocol simplifies decisions about how to sample controls, and it ensures that case-control differences in the risk factor of interest cannot be explained by reference to the matched variables. The disadvantages of matching include (1) it is time consuming and expensive; (2) some potential cases and controls may be excluded because matches cannot be made; (3) unmatched cases and controls must be discarded; (4) matched variables cannot be evaluated as risk factors in the study population; and (5) continuous matching categories may be too broad, and residual case control differences may persist.

Other types of case-control studies differ from population-based studies, primarily in the way the samples of cases and controls are selected. For convenience, a hospital-based study involves selection of hospital inpatients. In this type of study, the investigator selects cases (people admitted with the disease of interest to a particular hospital) and controls (people admitted with other conditions to the same hospital). Cases and controls are then interviewed in the hospital.

Hospital-based case-control studies can be very convenient because both the cases and the controls are found in the same institution. Potential subjects must not be too ill and must be willing to participate. Although hospital-based studies are convenient, they are also susceptible to distorted results. Cases and controls in a hospital may not arise from a single, well-defined population. These and related difficulties have led to a decline in popularity of hospital-based case-control studies.

The advantages of population-based samples for case-control study are that populations are better defined, it is easier to make certain that cases and controls derive from the same source population, and exposure histories of controls are more likely to reflect the people without the disease of interest. Hospital-based samples have subjects who are more accessible and cooperative, background characteristics of cases and controls that may be balanced, and an easier means to collect exposure information from medical records and biological specimens.

Data Analysis

Data collection and analysis are based on whether the case-control study involves a matched or unmatched design. The measure used typically in case-control studies is the odds ratio.

Odds ratio (OR): odds of a particular exposure among people with a specific condition divided by the corresponding odds of exposure among people without the condition under study; probability that a particular event will occur divided by the probability that the event will not occur; also called *relative odds*.

Unmatched Pair Design

The calculation of the odds ratio in an unmatched case-control design is as follows:

DISEASE STATUS

		Cases	Controls
	Present	A	B
EXPOSURE			
	Absent	C	D

$$OR = \frac{A \times D}{C \times B}$$

$$OR = \frac{\text{number of cases with exposure}}{\text{number of cases without exposure}} \times \frac{\text{number of controls without exposure}}{\text{number of controls with exposure}}$$

In this calculation, the cross-products of the entries in the 2 × 2 table are divided to arrive at the odds ratio. A cross-product is the multiplication of the diagonal entries or numbers. The number in cell A (number of exposed cases) is multiplied by the number in cell D (number of unexposed controls). The number in cell C (number of unexposed cases) is multiplied by the number in cell B (number of exposed controls). These two products are divided to arrive at the final result called an odds ratio.

Matched Pair Design

In this design, the number in each cell represents a pair (two people, one case subject and the matched control subject).

CONTROLS

		Exposure present	Exposure not present
	Exposure present	A	B
CASES			
	Exposure not present	C	D

$$OR = \frac{B}{C}$$

$$OR = \frac{\text{number of pairs in which only the case has been exposed} + \text{control has not been exposed}}{\text{number of pairs in which only the control has been exposed} + \text{case has not been exposed}}$$

In this study design, the calculation of the odds ratio takes into account the matched sampling scheme. Keep in mind that the entries, or numbers, in each cell consist of a pair of people that represent the relationship defined by that cell. In other words, in cell A above, the number presented would represent the number of matched pairs in which both the case-subject and the control-subject have been exposed. If the number were 5, that would mean that 5 matched pairs (of cases and controls, or a total of ten people) were exposed to the risk factor or variable under study. Calculation of the odds ratio in this design simply involves dividing the number in cell B (number of matched pairs in which the case is exposed but the control is not) by the number in cell C (number of matched pairs in which the case is not exposed but the control is exposed).

Cohort Study Design

A cohort study design usually consists of a prospective, observational, analytical study. It is an incidence study that is usually prospective or longitudinal and that measures attributes in a population free of the outcome of interest (e.g., disease, drug use) and relates them to subsequent development of the disease or outcome in that population as it is followed over time. This design is as close to an experimental approach as possible while still being observational in nature. It is used to study the risk of disease development.

There are many advantages to cohort studies. Direct calculation of the risk ratio or relative risk is possible. These studies provide information on incidence of disease and show temporal relationship between exposure and disease. They are appropriate for the study of rare exposures but not rare diseases. They provide information on multiple exposures and multiple outcomes for a particular exposure, and they minimize some biases. This design is the best observational one for establishing cause–effect relationships. Prevention and intervention measures can be tested and affirmed or rejected. Cohort studies take into account seasonal variation, fluctuations, or other changes over a longer period.

The disadvantages of cohort studies include that they are time consuming and expensive. They often require large sample sizes, and sampling problems can ensue. They are not efficient for the study of rare diseases. Losses to follow-up may diminish validity. Changes over time in diagnostic methods, exposures, or study population may lead to biased results. Locating subjects, developing tracking systems, and setting up examination and testing processes can be difficult. A disease outbreak or epidemic study has a very similar design to a cohort study, although it usually occurs over a much shorter timeframe.

Cohort studies are performed when intentional exposure of human beings cannot be justified. Cohort studies are observational because the investigator does not determine assignment of exposure but rather passively observes as exposures occur. Investigators follow the cohort over time to determine outcome(s) in exposed and unexposed subjects.

Selection of subjects for a cohort study is influenced by a variety of factors, including the type of exposure being investigated, the frequency of the exposure in the population, and the accessibility of subjects. Exposed and unexposed subjects must be free of the outcome of interest at the start of the study and equally susceptible to developing the outcome during the course of the study. If some subjects already have the outcome (e.g., disease) at the onset, then the temporal relationship between exposure and outcome becomes obscured.

The frequency of outcome occurrence in the exposed group of subjects is compared with the outcome frequency in the unexposed group of subjects. For this reason, it is essential to define the exposure clearly. Some exposures are acute, one-time episodes never repeated in a subject's lifetime. Other exposures are long term, such as cigarette smoking or use of oral contraceptives. Exposures may also be intermittent. Measurement of exposures should be based on intensity, duration, regularity, and variability. Guidelines for selection of exposed and unexposed subjects in a cohort study can include—

- Both exposed and unexposed subjects should be free of the disease of interest and equally susceptible to developing the disease at the beginning of the study.
- Information should be available on exposure and disease status in both groups.
- Both groups should be accessible and available for follow-up.
- Multiple comparison groups for exposed subjects chosen in different ways may reinforce the validity of findings.
- Objective measures of exposure, such as biological markers, are preferred over subjective measures.

Each subject must rigidly satisfy the criteria for inclusion in the cohort study, and he or she should not be excluded from subsequent analysis because of any change in exposure status during follow-up. The degree of surveillance should be similar in exposed and unexposed groups. Frequency of examination and duration of follow-up depend on the type of exposure and the outcome under investigation.

Occasionally, a cohort study is retrospective or historical in that it uses information on prior exposure and disease status. The advantage of the retrospective cohort design is that all of the events in the study have occurred and conclusions can be drawn more rapidly. Costs of a retrospective cohort study can be lower for the same reason. The retrospective approach also may be the only feasible one for studying effects from exposures that no longer occur, such as discontinued medical treatments. The main disadvantage of a retrospective cohort study is that the investigator must rely on existing records or subject recall.

A cohort may be open, meaning that subjects are allowed to enter the study at various times after it was started, or it may be closed, meaning that no subjects can be added to the study after it has begun. Analysis of open cohort data should use person-time units in the calculations. Person-time units are often used when individual subjects contribute across subcategories, such as age. For instance, a 48-year-old subject involved in a 5-year study would contribute 2 person-years to the 40- to 49-year-old group and 3 person-years to the 50- to 59-year-old group during the course of that study.

Following subjects over a long period of time can lead to a variety of problems. Dropouts and losses of subjects to follow-up are major problems in cohort studies. Subjects may move away or leave the study for other reasons, including deaths from other causes than the disease under investigation. If losses to follow-up are significant during the study, then the validity of the results can be seriously affected. It is also possible for exposure status to change during the course of the study. The exposure under study may be subject to variation over time. For example, cigarette smokers may quit, or employees may change jobs; therefore, their level of exposure to occupational hazards changes.

Midpoint analysis is used in cohort studies. A midpoint analysis occurs when, at a defined point in time in the study, all data collected to that point are analyzed so a decision can be made to stop or continue the study. Collection and analysis of data on the population subgroups, based on exposure, are divided according to variables of interest, like analysis in a cross-sectional study. Rates for subgroups are then calculated and compared. Finally, data from cohort studies are analyzed in terms of relative risk and attributable risk fractions.

Relative risk (RR): probability that a condition will occur; ratio of attack (AR) or other rates, such as incidence (IR); also called a risk ratio.

$$RR = \frac{AR \text{ (exposed group)}}{AR \text{ (unexposed group)}} \quad or \quad = \frac{IR \text{ (exposed group)}}{IR \text{ (unexposed group)}}$$

Attributable risk (AR): difference in rates between exposed group or group at risk (Re) and unexposed group (Rue).

$$AR = Re - Rue$$

Attributable risk fraction or percent (ARF or AR%): maximum proportion of a condition in a population that can be attributed to an etiological (causative) agent or other exposure or characteristic (risk factor); also proportional decrease in the incidence of a condition if the entire population were no longer exposed to the agent (risk factor).

$$ARF = \frac{Re - Rue}{Re}$$

Summary

The nature of the epidemiological investigation as well as the research questions posed dictate the choice of study design. Each design described in this chapter has its advantages and disadvantages and should be chosen based on the needs of, and constraints facing, the investigators. Future efforts in epidemiology will produce "hybrid" designs that further improve the classic study designs.

References

1. Lilienfeld DE, Stolley PD. *Foundations of Epidemiology*. 3rd ed. New York, NY: Oxford University Press; 1994.

2. Hennekens CH, Burning JE. *Epidemiology in Medicine*. Boston, Mass.: Little, Brown, and Co.; 1987.

3. Strom BL, Velo G, eds. *Drug Epidemiology and Post-Marketing Surveillance*. New York, NY: Plenum; 1992.

4. Marzuk PM, Tardiff K, Smyth D, Stajic M, Leon AC. Cocaine use, risk taking, and fatal Russian roulette. *JAMA*. 1992; 267:2635–2637.

Study Questions

1. In a cohort study, if subjects are added to the study after it has started, then the study is defined as a(n)—

    a. closed cohort study

    b. cross-sectional study

    c. open cohort study

    d. randomized controlled study

2. In a case-control study of exercise as a protective factor against development of osteoporosis, people with the disease (cases) tended to overestimate their level of exercise more than the control subjects. The likely effect of these overestimates on any observed relationship between the two variables is—

    a. to increase the apparent protective effect of exercise

    b. to decrease the apparent protective effect of exercise

    c. none

    d. impossible to predict from the information given

3. Match the epidemiological method with its corresponding description:

_____Case series study

_____Cross-sectional study

_____Case-control study

_____Cohort study

_____Clinical trial

a. an incidence study designed to assess attributes (variables) in a population and their relationship to the development of a condition or disease

b. an experimental design used to test the effectiveness of new treatments

c. a prevalence study designed to assess the occurrence of a condition or disease

d. a collection of separate reports on individual patients used to identify a potential problem

e. a retrospective study designed to determine causes of a disease

4. Define the following terms:

    a. descriptive study

    b. case report

    c. sampling

    d. case selection

    e. matching

    f. midpoint analysis

    g. loss to follow-up

5. Compare and contrast the following approaches:

    a. observational versus analytical epidemiology

    b. retrospective versus prospective designs

6. A prospective cohort study is conducted on the relationship between vitamin A use in the elderly and falls during nighttime. A total of 400 people age 50 years and older who use vitamin A daily are compared to a group of 400 people of same age who do not use vitamin A. Over a 1-year follow-up period, 20 vitamin A users suffer injuries from a fall that occurred after sunset, while 80 non–vitamin A users suffer injuries from nighttime falls. The attributable risk difference is—

    a. 0.05

    b. 0.10

    c. 0.15

    d. 0.20

    e. 0.50

The risk of nighttime fall attributable to nonuse of vitamin A (attributable risk percent) is—

    a. 15%

    b. 20%

    c. 50%

    d. 67%

    e. 75%

7. In a postmarketing surveillance study, you wish to assess the risk of a photosensitivity rash to users of your new antibiotic product. In a large health maintenance organization population, you identify 2194 users of your new antibiotic and 12,161 nonusers. During 1994, there were 28 new cases of photosensitivity rash in the user population and 53 cases of the rash in the nonuser population. Calculate the incidence rate (per 1000) of photosensitivity rash in each group and the relative risk of developing the rash if you were taking the new antibiotic product. What do you conclude?

8. A cohort study looks at the relationship between estrogen use and the risk of breast cancer. A total of 4555 estrogen users and 4495 nonusers are enrolled in the study and followed for 15 years for the development of breast cancer. In the estrogen-using group, 212 women develop breast cancer, and in the nonusing group, 298 women develop breast cancer. Calculate the risk of breast cancer in each group and the relative risk of developing breast cancer if a woman uses estrogen. Comment on your results.

9. The results of a 1979 case-control study assessing the risk of myocardial infarction (MI) based on use of oral contraceptive (OCs) are listed in Table 3-2 below. Calculate the overall (all ages) risk of MI based on use of OCs, and then calculate the risk for each age category. In which age category(ies) were women at greater risk for MI if they were using OCs? Comment briefly on the limitations of this type of method.

10. A 1992 case-control study (modified from Ref. 4) examined the association of alcohol and cocaine use as risk factors for suicide by Russian roulette (i.e., self-inflicted gunshot death). All of the control subjects were other drug-related deaths. Toxicological analyses were performed, and the data presented in Table 3-3 on the following page were obtained. What is the risk of death by Russian roulette compared with other drug-related deaths for alcohol and cocaine use?

TABLE 3-2. Data on Myocardial Infarction and Use of Oral Contraceptives

Age Group (years)	Exposure	Disease Status	
		MI	No Disease
25-29	Total number of women	7	356
	Number of women using OCs	2	108
30-34	Total number of women	11	371
	Number of women using OCs	4	119
35-39	Total number of women	9	306
	Number of women using OCs	3	85
40-44	Total number of women	26	396
	Number of women using OCs	9	97
45-49	Total number of women	41	423
	Number of women using OCs	18	112

Note: MI = Myocardial infarction; OC = oral contraceptive.

Name and describe at least one advantage and one disadvantage in the use of this epidemiological method to test the research question, whether alcohol or cocaine use influences the risk of committing suicide by Russian roulette.

TABLE 3-3. **Data on Alcohol and Cocaine Use and Risk of Suicide**

	Suicide by Russian Roulette	*Other Drug-Related Deaths*	*Totals*
Alcohol present	11	33	44
Alcohol absent	3	21	24
Totals	14	54	68
Cocaine present	14	23	37
Cocaine absent	5	45	50
Totals	19	68	87

Chapter 4

Experimental Study Designs

Experimental study designs are the primary method for testing the effectiveness of new therapies and other interventions, including innovative drugs. By the 1930s, the pharmaceutical industry had adopted experimental methods and other research designs to develop and screen new compounds, improve production outputs, and test drugs for therapeutic benefits. The full potential of experimental methods in drug research was realized in the 1940s and 1950s with the growth in scientific knowledge and industrial technology.[1]

In the 1960s, the controlled clinical trial, in which a group of patients receiving an experimental drug is compared with another group receiving a control drug or no treatment, became the standard for doing pharmaceutical research and measuring the therapeutic benefits of new drugs.[1] By the same time, the double-blind strategy of drug testing, in which both the patients and the researcher are unaware of which treatment is being taken by whom, had been adopted to limit the effect of external influences on the true pharmacological action of the drug. The drug regulations of the 1960s also reinforced the importance of controlled clinical trials by requiring that proof of effectiveness for new drugs be made through use of these research methods.[2,3]

In pharmacoepidemiology, the primary use of experimental design is in performing clinical trials, most notably randomized, controlled clinical trials.[4] These studies involve people as the units of analysis. A variation on this experimental design is the community intervention study, in which groups of people, such as whole communities, are the unit of analysis. Key aspects of the clinical and community intervention trial designs are randomization, blinding, intention-to-treat analysis, and sample size determination.

Experimental Design

An *experiment* is a study designed to compare benefits of an intervention with standard treatments, or no treatment, such as a new drug therapy or prevention program, or to show cause and effect (see Figure 3-2). This type of study is performed prospectively. Subjects are selected from a study population, assigned to the various study groups, and monitored over time to determine the outcomes that occur and are produced by the new drug therapy, treatment, or intervention.

Experimental designs have numerous advantages compared with other epidemiological methods. Randomization, when used, tends to balance confounding variables across the various study groups, especially variables that might be associated with changes in the disease state or the outcome of the intervention under study. Detailed information and data are collected at the beginning of an experimental study to develop a baseline; this same type of information also is collected at specified follow-up periods throughout the study. The investigators have control over variables such as the dose or degree of intervention. The blinding process reduces distortion in assessment. And, of great value, and not possible with other methods, is the testing of hypotheses. Most important, this design is the only real test of cause–effect relationships.

The disadvantages of experimental design involve subject participation criteria that may limit generalizability of findings. Restrictive criteria for inclusion or exclusion of subjects may produce a very homogeneous study population that restricts application of the results to patients with other characteristics. Clinical trials, especially those focused on chronic diseases, may require years of follow-up and prolonged observation to determine treatment outcomes. The result is often higher costs, increased likelihood that patients will be lost to follow-up, and delayed treatment recommendations. Large sample sizes are typically required to demonstrate differences among study groups, especially if there is wide variability in responses to treatment. Increasing the size of the study population also raises the cost of the trial and may make it difficult to locate a sufficiently large pool of eligible patients. Ethical concerns also arise in clinical trials, and subjects may not comply with the treatment and assignment.

Clinical trials can be divided into three types: (1) therapeutic trials in which therapeutic agents or procedures are given to patients in an attempt to cure the disease, relieve symptoms, or prolong survival; (2) intervention trials in which the investigator intervenes before the disease has developed in individuals with certain characteristics that increase their risk of developing the disease; and (3) prevention trials in which an attempt is made to determine the efficacy of a preventive agent or procedure among people who do not have the disease but may be at greater risk for developing it. The randomized, controlled clinical trial is the most widely accepted approach for comparing the benefits of treatments. The basic design of a randomized, controlled clinical trial is outlined in Figure 4-1. Community intervention trials have the same basic design; the difference is that groups of people are assigned to the various study groups.

Clinical Drug Trials

Recall from the first chapter of this book the description of James Lind's study aimed at finding a treatment for scurvy. His study with the sailors is an example of the direct comparison of two or more treatments in human beings who have the same disease—what is known today as a clinical trial. The development of the clinical trial

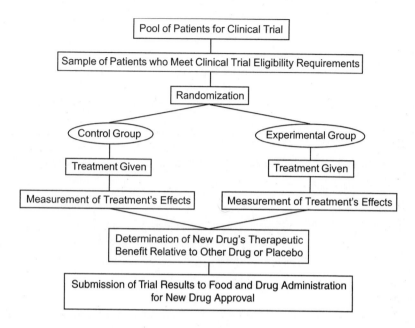

Figure 4-1. Randomized, controlled clinical trial.

is a product of the application of the modern scientific method to medicine. Experiments on human populations, however, have inherent difficulties not found in the laboratory. Whereas laboratory experiments involve controlled environments and the manipulation of just a small number of variables, control of human subjects and their environments, with a variety of other factors, is much more difficult.

The many types of contemporary drug trials use a variety of approaches. The basic idea is to "try out" (trial) a new drug in clinical practice on sick patients. The goal is to determine the therapeutic benefits of the new drug in humans after it has passed safety testing in animals as well as safety, dosage range, and effectiveness studies. These requirements are known as phases I and II in drug development. As outlined in Table 4-1, the design of drug trials varies by certain components: the specific treatments being evaluated and compared, how patients are selected for the different study groups, and who knows which patients are receiving the experimental treatment and which ones are receiving other treatments or no treatment.

Clinical drug trials also vary considerably in their design features. There is "clinical inquiry," a simple, nonexperimental method in which only one group of patients receives a new drug, and data are collected and analyzed to see if it had any effect; no control or comparison group is used. In the controlled clinical trial, the control group consists of participants not from the original pool of potential study patients or patients whose past cases involved receiving other treatments in regular health care or research situations. In other words, a controlled trial may not include the process of random assignment of all patients into the different treatment groups.

TABLE 4-1. **Components of a Clinical Drug Trial**

Experimental study: A research method in which one group of subjects receives a new treatment (e.g., drug, device, surgery), and they are compared with one or more other group(s) who receive different standard treatments or placebo. These groups are studied over the same time period using the same measures of safety and effectiveness.

Experimental group: The group of patients that receives the drug under investigation.

Control group: The group of patients that receives a different type of treatment, either a traditional one (already approved and used in therapy) or no treatment (a placebo).

Randomization: The process of assigning individual patients to different treatment groups in such a way that each patient has the same chance, equal to and independent of every other patient, of being selected for any particular study or treatment group. The idea is to make all study groups as equal as possible at the beginning of the experiment.

Blinding: The process of ensuring that almost everyone involved in the drug trial is unaware of who is receiving the experimental drug and who is receiving a traditional drug treatment, or a placebo, throughout the duration of the study. In experimental studies, lack of knowledge about which patients are receiving which treatments may be limited to the patients (single-blind); patients and treating clinicians (double-blind); or patients, treating clinicians, and the scientific investigators (triple-blind).

Placebo: An inactive form of treatment, usually an inert sugar pill, received by patients in the control group. This treatment provides the basis for a trial group (the controls) to receive no (beneficial) treatment so that a good comparison can be made with the results of the experimental group. The use of placebo in most clinical trials is declining due to ethical concerns.

The best method for determining the true therapeutic benefit of a new unknown treatment is the randomized, controlled clinical trial. Today, a clinical trial is often performed at more than one facility. These multisite studies may link together a number of hospitals, clinics, and research centers to increase the number and diversity of the subjects who choose to participate in it, leading to more powerful and generalizable results. This feature may also shorten the time of the study.

Randomized, Controlled Clinical Trials

Few people would argue today that the most scientific and ethical method for investigation of new therapies is the randomized, controlled clinical trial. The main objective of this method is to make certain that, after the trial is over, the better (or best) of the studied treatments is identified. The key components in a randomized clinical trial is the use of a control group and randomization of subjects into the study groups (see Table 4-1). Not all clinical trials, however, are of this type.

In some circumstances, the randomization process may not be justified. This issue has arisen in recent research on drugs for treatment of AIDS. Patients with AIDS believe that they all should be in the clinical trial and in the new investigational drug study group. No one should be denied an experimental treatment because they were randomly selected to be in the control or placebo group. Regardless of whether a randomization process is justified in a particular drug study, patients should always be informed of any randomization process that is being used to influence their treatment choices.

Although there has been much progress in the design and conduct of clinical trials, they still are far from being a perfect method. The clinical drug trial may be thought of as a large-scale, standardized alternative to the process whereby individual clinicians gradually accumulate knowledge through direct clinical experience with a particular therapy. Clinical trials answer only questions that have been asked specifically. One argument concerning the usefulness of clinical trials is that the experimental conditions of the trial often differ so much from the conditions encountered in clinical practice that the trial's results may not be applicable to real-life situations. Concerns about the quality of clinical trials are another issue.

Randomization

Randomization is a key aspect of clinical trials. It maximizes the probability that the two groups are as similar as possible in terms of background characteristics, especially factors and variables that may influence response to therapy or primary outcome measure. In a randomized study, treatment group assignment is based on probability alone and is not influenced by the physicians' or patients' preferences.

Mathematics and the law of probability also influence how clinical trials are done and why the randomization process is needed. Every patient in the original patient pool, or group, must have a chance equal to every other patient of being assigned to a particular treatment group. For instance, what if in a study of a new pain medication, the investigators decided to take the first 25 patients who were interested in participating and assign them to the experimental (new pain medication) group. The next 25 patients who were interested were assigned to the control (placebo) group. What would the study results mean if the investigators found that the new pain medication was significantly more effective than the placebo?

It could be that the first 25 patients were those with a greater degree of pain. Patients heard about the clinical trial, and those hurting the most went to see the investigators sooner than those patients with less pain. This circumstance makes for a difference between the two groups, in terms of their pain experience, from the beginning of the study, before anyone began taking the new drug. This situation would not set up a good comparison for the new drug because the group receiving it was sicker than the control or comparison group before the trial began. The drug could seem to be more, or even less, effective than it really is when the comparison is made.

Blinding

Blinding, or masking, is a process of keeping individuals involved in the study unaware of assignment of subjects to different study groups. *Single-blind* means keeping the subjects unaware; *double-blind* means keeping the investigators and subjects unaware; and there is even a *triple-blind* study, in which data analysis is done by outside evaluators independent of the investigators.

When a study is double-blinded and randomization of patients was used, most people involved in the study should not know who is getting which treatment, or no treatment, and a more objective assessment of the new therapy can be made. Of course, the blinding process can break down in studies where some patients are not receiving any treatment, and other patients are taking a very active drug with intensely noticeable, specific effects. In this instance, it will only be a short time during the study before patients begin to realize who is getting the drug, based on the significant effects that some of the patients are experiencing.

Intention-to-Treat and Interim Analyses

Intention-to-treat analysis involves comparison of the entire experimental group with the entire study group(s) regardless of whether subjects in those groups completed the full course of their study treatments. Analyses are based on the first observations recorded on subjects, which is usually connected to their initial treatment assignments. As in cohort studies, loss to follow-up is an issue in clinical trials. Although this issue represents a major bias in cohort studies, investigators often have more control over patient involvement throughout the clinical trial because of the patient's investment in seeking a new, better treatment. In both study designs, the key issue is whether the probability of loss to follow-up is related to exposures, treatments, the disease, and other study outcomes. The major advantage of intention-to-treat analysis is that it maintains the randomization scheme, as subjects do not randomly drop out of studies.

In the design of a clinical trial, it is necessary to develop guidelines for deciding whether a trial should be modified or stopped before originally scheduled. This decision is usually based on interim analyses. In some trials of preventive and therapeutic regimens, individuals may be under study over an extended period, and the experiences of early participants become available while other individuals are still being enrolled in the study. To ensure that the welfare of the participants is protected, and to provide useful new therapies to the medical community, available study result should be monitored at various points, arguably by a group that is independent of the investigators conducting the trial. If the data indicate a clearly significant benefit in terms of the primary endpoint, or if one treatment is clearly harmful, then early termination of the trial must be considered.

The decision to terminate a study early is based on a number of complex issues and must be made with great caution. A method for monitoring the accumulating data from a clinical trial is necessary, and a general rule must be in place for assessment. The first requirement for considering termination or modification is the observation of a sustained statistical association that is extreme and highly significant, virtually impossible to arise by chance alone. Statistical test results should not be used, however, as the sole basis for the decision to stop or continue a trial. Those tests serve an important function—to alert the investigators to consider taking action. Observing significant associations must be considered in the context of the totality of evidence, including postulated or known biological mechanisms that might explain the results, the results of other clinical trials or observational studies, and assessment of how the observed associations relate to an overall risk-to-benefit ratio of the treatment.

Process of Performing a Clinical Trial

There are a number of steps in the process, or protocol, for performing a clinical trial (see Table 4-2). The first step in performing a clinical trial, as in any

TABLE 4-2. **Process (Protocol) for Designing a Clinical Trial**

State research question or hypothesis.

State rationale and background for study.

Determine endpoints or outcomes for study.

Select study design (including blinding, randomization, types and durations of treatments, and number of patients).

Describe selection process for study population and state criteria for including and excluding subjects.

Outline treatment procedures.

Define all clinical, laboratory, and other tests.

Determine methods for ensuring integrity of the data.

Develop procedures for handling side effects and problem cases.

Develop procedures for obtaining informed consent.

Develop procedures for periodic review of trial data and termination of trial.

Randomize patients to experimental and control groups.

Compare treatment groups regarding baseline factors.

Perform follow-up on (monitor) patients, including interim analyses.

Determine number of patients involved in final results and lost to follow-up (intention-to-treat analysis).

Calculate rates and confidence intervals for study data.

Report nature and number of side effects and other problems.

Assess data and results in light of study question or hypothesis.

experiment, is to formulate the major research question. This question usually is referred to as a *hypothesis*. The research question determines the importance of selected independent variables, such as the types of interventions or treatments to be compared and the nature of the dependent variables, endpoints, or outcomes to be evaluated.

Additional aspects in the early stages of a trial include the number and nature of subjects for the study as well as eligibility and exclusion requirements for subject participation in the study. Endpoints must be determined in terms of clinical importance, which ones can be measured in a reasonable manner, and which ones can be studied in the given population with the constraints and resources available to the study. More than one endpoint can be measured to assess treatment efficacy. Examples of specific endpoints include measures of the quality of life, length of survival, percentage of patients surviving, remission or hospitalization rates, and the proportion of patients with recurring symptoms or complications.

Sample Size Determination and Data Analysis

The number of subjects who should be enrolled in the clinical trial is known as the *sample size*. This number should be determined soon after the primary research question or outcome has been formulated. At the conclusion of an experiment, the data are analyzed and a statistical decision is made either to accept or to reject the hypothesis.

The decision to accept or reject a hypothesis is based on probabilities, and the study results based on these decisions may not truly reflect what is occurring in "reality." Reality, or "the truth," can be thought of as the results of the intervention when they are applied correctly to all possible patients (i.e., anyone with the clinical condition). The clinical trial results can be thought of as one sample of the truth, or reality. Using only a sample of the entire patient population for the trial, the investigator hopes to use the trial's results to generalize about all patients. The problem is that the investigator is intervening only on the study sample and cannot intervene with the whole population of patients. There is always a risk of arriving at a mistaken conclusion because the trial sample did not represent all types of patients with the same disease.

Consider an example showing the relationship between clinical trial results and reality. Cells A and D represent a relationship between study results and reality that is correct. The study results are valid and truly reflect what would happen to other patients in the population if they were given the same treatment as those in the trial sample. In cell A, the study results and reality both indicate that the outcomes are different (e.g., the new drug is more effective than a placebo). This is also known as a *true-positive result*. In cell D, the study results and reality both indicate that the outcomes are not different (e.g., the new drug is not more effective than a placebo). This is known as a *true-negative result*.

REALITY

		Outcome different	Outcome not different
		A	B
	Outcome different	Study result valid (true positive)	Type I error (false positive)
STUDY RESULTS		C	D
	Outcome Not different	Type II error (false negative)	Study result valid (true negative)

Two types of errors can be made in interpreting study results. The results might indicate that there is a difference in outcomes or treatments when in reality there is no difference (cell B). This is a type I error; under these circumstances, the study results are not valid but are falsely positive. For the other type of error, if the study failed to find a difference in outcomes or treatments when there actually was a difference, a type II error has occurred (cell C); under these circumstances, the study results are not valid but are falsely negative.

Falsely positive or falsely negative study results can occur because of faulty methodology, chance occurrence, or for both reasons. Although some errors can be minimized by careful attention to study design, errors due to chance can never be completely eliminated. Such errors, however, can be estimated. The notation used to describe the likelihood of a type I error (i.e., the difference observed between treatment groups is not a true difference but due instead to chance) is the *alpha* (α) *level*. The notation used to describe the likelihood of a type II error (i.e., the study did not find a difference between treatment groups when there is indeed a difference) is called the *beta* (β) *level*. Researchers specify α and β levels when planning a study. For instance, an α level may be specified at 0.05, which means the investigator is willing to accept a 5% risk of committing a type I error, falsely concluding that the treatment groups differ when in reality they do not. Likewise, the investigator may specify a β level, or risk of committing a type II error, of 0.1. In other words, a 10% chance of missing a true difference between the treatment groups is being allowed.

The *statistical power*, or ability of a study to detect a true difference between groups, is $1-\beta$. Thus, for a β level of 0.10, the study would have a 90% chance of detecting the true difference in outcomes between treatment groups. Once the α and β levels have been established, the investigator must specify another extremely important study parameter for determining sample size—the magnitude of the difference in outcome between treatment groups that the study will be designed to detect. This difference between treatments under comparison is of great importance and should be selected on the basis of clinical information. In deciding on the level of outcome difference for detection, the following may be considered: (1) the difference in outcome that would be important to clinicians treating this type of patient, (2) the difference that would be meaningful to a patient who may suffer the consequences of the disease, and (3) the difference in outcome that would justify use of the more effective treatment despite greater expense or greater side effects.

Data analysis in clinical trials is based on the research question(s) and outcome measures, but typically some form of rate is calculated. Data analysis can be simple (e.g., the comparative outcome in the trial is only the mortality rate) or complex, employing multivariate statistics and many different analyses to determine differences in outcomes.

Clinical Trials and the U.S. Drug Approval Process

There are four major steps in the U.S. drug development and approval process (see Figure 4-2). Drug development begins with the preliminary development and identification of potentially useful compounds through preclinical research. Compounds that show promise and a pharmaceutical company wishes to explore are approved for further study, clinical testing, by the U.S. Food and Drug Administration (FDA). Clinical testing occurs in four phases, three of which take place before the drug is approved for the market; the fourth occurs in postmarketing. The final step of drug development involves review and approval of the drug and marketing it to the public.[1]

Step 1: Preliminary Development (Preclinical Research)

Initial discovery and synthesis of a new chemical compound are the beginnings of preclinical research toward the marketing of a prescription drug. Discovery of an effective and safe drug may involve hundreds of chemical structures and molecular formulas that are initially considered before one becomes a truly useful prescription drug. Evaluation of a potential new drug begins in the laboratories of pharmaceutical manufacturers and occurs in animals. Both short-term (1 to 3 years) and long-term (2 to 10 years) research are conducted to determine safety and efficacy of a new compound. Hundreds of compounds are synthesized, developed, and researched in this manner each year, compared with the 20 to 30 new drugs that are approved by the FDA annually.

Step 2: Filing an Investigational New Drug Application (with 30-Day Wait Period)

After successful laboratory and animal tests with a new compound, the second step is submission of an investigational new drug (IND) application to the FDA. An investigational new drug is a new pharmaceutical product that has not been shown to be safe and effective in humans but that seems to be safe and effective in the management of a disease or condition on the basis of animal tests. An IND is submitted by a pharmaceutical manufacturer to the FDA to request permission to conduct clinical trials of the drug in humans. After a 30-day, IND-review period, the sponsor is allowed to investigate the clinical value of the drug. If there are any concerns regarding the drug's safety, the FDA places the IND on clinical hold, and the sponsor may not begin testing until changes are made to eliminate safety concerns.

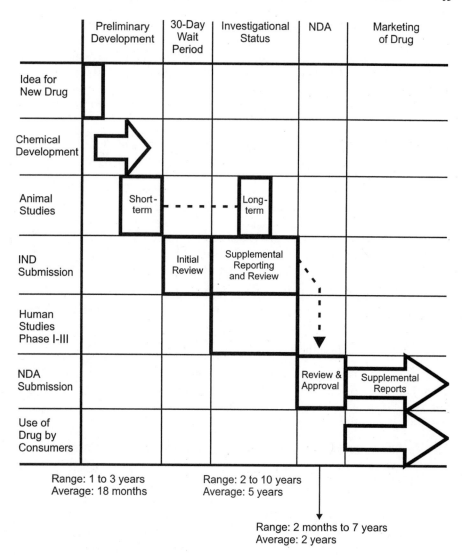

Figure 4-2. The U.S. drug approval process. (IND = investigational new drug; NDA = new drug application.) (*Source:* U.S. Food and Drug Administration.)

Step 3: Clinical Testing of Investigational New Drug

Unless the FDA puts an IND on clinical hold during the review period, clinical testing of the drug can begin. The overall goal is to collect and review data to determine whether the possibility of adverse events outweighs the expected usefulness of the drug. Before marketing, clinical trials are conducted in three phases.

Phase I: Clinical Pharmacology and Toxicology. The first phase of clinical testing is directed at determining the drug's safe dosage range, the preferred administration route, the mechanisms of absorption and distribution in the body, and possible toxicities. These tests usually are conducted in a small number (20 to 80) normal healthy volunteers and require less than 12 months to complete. A majority (50% to 70%) of compounds tested in phase I are abandoned due to problems with safety.

Phase II: Initial Clinical Efficacy and Tolerability. The purpose of phase II is to learn more about the drug's safety and efficacy in treating a certain disease or symptom. These studies also use a small number (50 to 200) of volunteers who have the disease or symptom for which the drug seems to be effective. Additional animal testing also can occur during phase II to gain further information about the drug's long-term safety. Phase II trials usually require up to 2 years. If the studies show that the drug is useful in a particular disease and animal data show no unwarranted harm, then the sponsor can proceed to phase III. According to the FDA, approximately one third of new drugs continue on to phase III.

Phase III: Treatment Efficacy. The third phase of clinical trials involves the most extensive drug testing. Phase III studies assess safety, efficacy, and appropriate dosage range for the drug in treating a specific disease in a large group of patients. The number of patients involved can range from several hundred to several thousand, depending on the drug. During phase III studies, the drug is used by practicing physicians in a manner similar to the way in which it would be used when marketed. Additional testing to characterize more specifically the adverse effects of the drug is also conducted in phase III. On average, only about 25% of new drugs successfully pass through phase III testing.

Step 4: Review and Approval of the New Drug Application and Marketing

After clinical testing of the new drug, the manufacturer is required to submit a new drug application (NDA) to the FDA. The NDA review and approval process usually requires 2 to 3 years. The NDA review and approval process nears completion when the FDA sends the drug's sponsor an approval letter. A supplemental new drug application (supplemental NDA) is submitted when a drug's sponsor requests approval to promote an existing drug with either a new indication or new labeling or when manufacturing procedures have changed. Because the same regulations and requirements do not apply for review and approval of a supplemental NDA as for a standard NDA, the request does not undergo the same scope of review and is approved more quickly.

Phase IV: Postmarketing Surveillance. After a drug is approved and released to the market, the sponsor (e.g., pharmaceutical company) must continue to submit information to the FDA on a regular basis. Such data requirements are considered phase IV clinical trials and are a part of postmarketing surveillance of the drug product. Since the early 1970s, the FDA has been responsible for monitoring the safety and quality of drugs on the market. Another part of phase IV studies involves clinical trials of the drug in various subgroups of patients, such as children or women.

Patient Compliance in Clinical Drug Research

The failure of patients to take drugs as prescribed, called *noncompliance*, has been documented, and its implications for patient care are well known to health professionals. The impact noncompliance can have on the drug development process, from clinical trials to marketing, has not been well appreciated by pharmaceutical manufacturers and regulators. Noncompliance occurs for a variety of reasons, and many determinants have been identified through research.

Noncompliance by participants in clinical trials affects the evaluation and approval of new pharmaceutical agents at two stages. First, during the pre-approval drug development phases, noncompliance may alter results of clinical investigations that determine the optimal dose for package insert labeling. After the drug has been approved and is marketed, noncompliance, especially if it is widespread, may lead to the emergence of unexpected problems, such as irregular dosing, overprescribing, failures to achieve patient care outcomes, and toxicities.

Some drug approval delays can be attributed to noncompliance and the failure of clinical investigators to recognize it. There may be difficulty in demonstrating a drug's effectiveness in intention-to-treat analyses, which assumes that patients follow the regimens to which they were assigned. Noncompliance also can interfere with determination of therapeutic dosage ranges. Most trials that now report the safety and efficacy of a drug do not reflect the individual patient's response to a prescribed dosage. They reflect a composite of the responses of patients who fail to comply, those who partially comply, and those who fully comply with the therapeutic regimen.

Adjustments for noncompliance in analysis of clinical trial data might be in opposition to the intention-to-treat approach, although noncompliant patients can complete an entire study. It is necessary to take into account the impact of known compliance or noncompliance on estimates of a drug's safety and efficacy. Giving equal weight to compliant patients who took the drug and to patients who never took the drug, took the wrong drug, or took inadequate amounts increases the probability of overestimating the therapeutic dose range. Adverse reactions then could occur when patients take the recommended dose in practice. Additional trials may be necessary for approval, and the problem resides with patient noncompliance, not the drug product's dose or formulation. Noncompliance also affects statistical analysis of clinical trial and postmarketing data.

Clinical trial research, particularly on chronic diseases, must include new endpoints. Priority should be given to subjective, in addition to objective, endpoints that imply a focus on risk factors and symptomatic treatments over cures. Such research needs to emphasize the psychosocial component as equally or more important than the biological component. These areas of study are exploring the emergent quality-of-life concepts and new ethical priorities in health care.

Summary

It should be obvious that clinical drug trials, especially the randomized, controlled type, are an excellent approach for determining the actual beneficial effects of new drug compounds.

The clinical drug trial may be thought of as a large-scale, standardized alternative to the process whereby individual clinicians gradually accumulate knowledge through bedside clinical experience with a particular therapy. In essence, clinical medicine is made scientific through clinical trials. In a drug trial, clinical observations tend to be made in a systematic manner, whereas, in personal clinical experience, they tend to be anecdotal. Personal experience is usually more subjective and less quantitative, or numerical, than observations based on a randomized, controlled experimental design. In contrast, clinical trials answer only the questions that have been specifically asked. Personal experience can take into account factors that have not yet been examined in the trial process.

A recent development has been the multisite clinical trial, which is an experiment that involves two or more clinical facilities, each of which is responsible for recruitment, treatment, and follow-up of patients under a commonly agreed plan. Data and information from all of the centers is combined in the research analysis stage. Multisite trials have a number of advantages. The majority of single trials that are performed have too few patients and usually lack ethnic diversity of subjects, so a multisite approach can greatly increase the number of participants in the study. Such trials, however, can be more complex to organize and operate as well as more costly to run. Not only do these trials have the potential for recruiting adequate numbers of patients, but the range of different people involved also usually leads to a better research design and more careful execution of the study. The larger number of clinics and the different patient populations also may provide a more realistic test of the treatment in question.

References

1. Basara LR, Montagne M. *Searching for Magic Bullets: Orphan Drugs, Consumer Activism and Pharmaceutical Development*. Binghamton, NY: Haworth Press; 1994.

2. Guarino RA, ed. *New Drug Approval Process*. 2nd ed. New York, NY: Marcel Dekker; 1993.

3. Lilienfeld DE, Stolley PD. *Foundations of Epidemiology*. 3rd ed. New York, NY: Oxford University Press; 1994.

4. Strom BL, Velo G, eds. *Drug Epidemiology and Post-Marketing Surveillance*. New York, NY: Plenum; 1992.

Study Questions

1. The assessment of study data based on initial assignments to treatment groups, regardless of whether the subjects completed a full course of the treatments, is called—

    a. midpoint analysis

    b. randomization

    c. intention-to-treat analysis

    d. validity

2. The purpose of randomization in a controlled clinical trial is—

    a. to obtain treatment groups of similar size

    b. to select a representative sample from the population

    c. to increase patient compliance with the treatments

    d. to obtain treatment groups with similar baseline characteristics

3. All randomized, controlled clinical trials involve the use of a placebo group.

    a. true

    b. false

4. Define the following terms:

    a. experimental design

    b. community intervention study

    c. clinical trials

    d. randomized, controlled clinical trial

    e. randomization

    f. blinding

    g. sample size determination

5. In a clinical trial, 9 of 29 asthmatics taking a new drug continue to have asthma attacks 3 months later, whereas 12 of 74 asthmatics using a new breathing exercise continue to have asthma attacks. Which new treatment approach is more effective in preventing asthma attacks?

6. A study was begun in 1975 to assess the effectiveness of aspirin in preventing recurrent myocardial infarctions (MIs) in individuals who have survived an MI. It was a multisite, randomized, double-blind, placebo-controlled study. Aspirin was given to patients in one study group (the experimental group), and mortality was assessed over a 3-year period. Eligible patients were men and women, 30 through 69 years of age, who had had at least one MI. Exclusion criteria included individuals with aspirin intolerance, ulcer disease, previous cardiovascular surgery, uncontrolled hypertension, and medication use that included aspirin or drugs that interacted with aspirin. Endpoints, or outcome measures, were fatal and nonfatal MI, stroke, or other cardiovascular event. Study enrollment was 4524 patients; 2267 were randomized to the experimental group (1 gram aspirin/day), and 2257 were randomized to the control (placebo) group. Major results are presented in Table 4-3 below. Calculate the relative risk of another MI for each set of rates presented in the data table. What recommendations would you make to the medical community?

TABLE 4-3. **Data on Aspirin's Effectiveness in Preventing Recurrent MI**

Outcome	Aspirin Group (%)	Placebo Group (%)
Total mortality rate	10.8	9.7
Coronary mortality rate	8.7	8.0
Cardiovascular mortality rate	0.6	0.7
Noncardiovascular mortality rate	1.4	0.9
Mortality rate, men over 175 pounds	11.0	9.6
Mortality rate, women under 144 pounds	7.6	4.3
Mortality rate, women over 144 pounds	8.3	6.1

Chapter 5

Data Identification and Analysis

During the design phase of a study, the investigator must decide which type of data will be collected and analyzed. Large amounts of data will be collected, and not all of the data can or will be reported in the published account. The investigator must decide how to most appropriately summarize and present the large volume of data collected to give readers an accurate understanding of the study results.

It is important to be able to differentiate between various types of data. The type of data collected will determine how the data are presented, described, and analyzed.[1,2] Just as there are multiple types of data, there are various methods of describing and summarizing data. These methods are referred to as *descriptive methods*. After the data are described and summarized, the data are analyzed statistically using inferential methods. Whereas descriptive methods simply describe or summarize data, inferential methods are used to make inferences about populations. This chapter discusses the various types of data, explains the most common means with which data are described and summarized, and introduces inferential methods.

Types of Data

There are two types of data: discrete and continuous. It is important to be able to differentiate between the two because the type of data that is collected determines how the data are reported and analyzed. *Discrete data* fit into a limited number of categories and are also referred to as *count data*. Each subject fits into only one discrete category.

The simplest form of discrete data is a dichotomous variable. Dichotomous variables have only two categories per variable. An example of a dichotomous variable is gender. Each subject in a study is either male or female. There are only two options or categories possible for this dichotomous variable. Other examples of dichotomous variables include questions that would be answered with a yes or a no. For example, an investigator may wish to solicit information from subjects about whether they have any significant past medical history. Subjects would be given a list of several medical conditions (e.g., hypertension, hypercholesterolemia, myocardial infarction) and asked to answer yes or no to having been diagnosed with each condition.

If the discrete data have more than two possible values or categories, then they are referred to as multichotomous. Race is an example of a multichotomous discrete variable. Race can be divided into many possible categories: black, white, Asian, Hispanic, and so forth.

Another type of discrete variable is an ordinal variable. Ordinal variables have a limited number of values or categories, but the categories are in a logical order or progression. An example of an ordinal variable is degree of inflammation. When data on degree of inflammation are collected, it is typically measured in +1, +2, or +3 categories. In this case, +1 inflammation is the mildest form, and +3 is the most severe form of inflammation. Similar scales are often used to measure pain. An investigator may ask a subject to report his or her pain on a scale of 1 to 5, with 1 being the least pain and 5 being the worst pain.

Continuous data can take on any number of values along a specified continuum. Unlike discrete data, continuous data do not fit into a finite number of categories. Continuous data are often referred to as *measurement data*. An example of a continuous variable is age, which can be measured in units of days, weeks, months, or years. Other examples of continuous variables are weight, height, and blood pressure. Any measurements made from the blood or urine (e.g., serum drug levels, serum creatinine, serum electrolytes, urine drug levels) can be considered to be continuous variables.

It is important to note that many variables can be treated as either discrete or continuous. Again, age is an example. Age can be treated as a continuous variable and measured in units of days or years. When measured, age can assume any value along a continuum that begins at day 1 and ends somewhere near 100 years. Table 5-1 displays a data set of 10 subjects and the corresponding age of each subject. In

TABLE 5-1. Age Reported as a Continuous Variable

Subject	Age (years)
1	21
2	26
3	29
4	35
5	36
6	43
7	49
8	50
9	55
10	59

TABLE 5-2. Age Reported as a
Discrete Variable

Age as a Discrete Variable (years)	Number of Subjects
20–29	3
30–39	2
40–49	2
50–59	3

this example, age is treated as a continuous variable. Table 5-2, however, displays age as a discrete variable. When age is treated as a discrete variable, a finite number of age categories is created such that each subject fits into only one category.

Most studies involve multiple measurements on each subject at various points. For example, if an investigator is studying the effects of an antihypertensive medication on blood pressure, then blood pressure measurement will be made at baseline (before the intervention) and at various times after the treatment has begun (e.g., every 4 weeks for 6 months). The investigator must decide whether to analyze the results using paired or unpaired statistical methods. Paired methods analyze the difference between two measurements or observations. Paired analyses are most commonly used to analyze before and after results. Unpaired analyses involve analysis of only one measurement or observation per subject, whereas unpaired analyses most commonly analyze the end result. Both continuous and discrete data can be considered to be either paired or unpaired.

Distribution of Data

Once data are collected, they are typically plotted on a distribution curve. The simplest distribution curve plots one variable along the x-axis and the number of subjects along the y-axis. Data can assume distribution curves that are either normally distributed or skewed. In a normal distribution, all observations are clustered around the middle of the curve. The distribution is symmetrical, and the curve is bell-shaped. A normal distribution is also referred to as a *Gaussian distribution* or a *parametric distribution*. Figure 5-1 depicts a normal distribution of weight in a given population. Weight is reported on the x-axis, and the number of subjects is indicated on the y-axis.

Not all data assume a normal distribution when plotted. Data can also appear as a skewed distribution. Skewed distributions are also referred to as *non-Gaussian* or *nonparametric distributions*. In a skewed distribution, data are not clustered around the middle, and the distribution is not symmetrical. In a skewed distribution, data will be clustered at one of the two tails of the distribution curve. Skewed data can be positively or negatively skewed. Positively skewed data, or data in which the tail of the distribution is skewed to the right, have the majority of

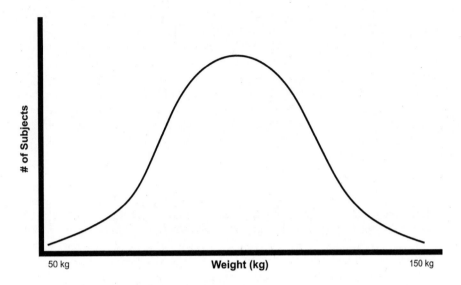

Figure 5-1. Normal distribution of weight.

observations occurring at the lower end of the x-axis of the distribution curve. Negatively skewed data, or data in which the tail of the distribution is skewed to the left, will have the majority of observations occurring at the higher end of the x-axis. Figure 5-2 represents a weight distribution that is skewed to the left, and Figure 5-3 represents a weight distribution that is skewed to the right.

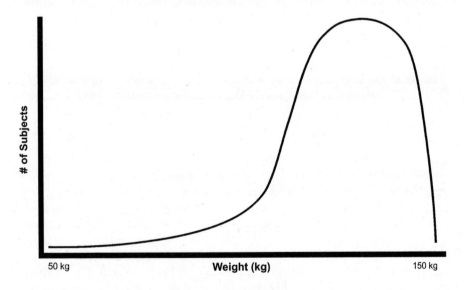

Figure 5-2. Weight distribution skewed to the left.

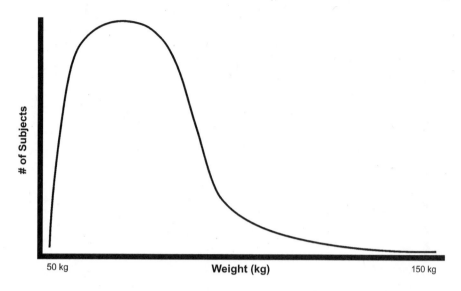

Figure 5-3. Weight distribution skewed to the right.

Measures of Central Tendency

Several measures of central tendency are used to describe data sets. These measures are often referred to as *descriptive statistics*. Descriptive statistics is an effective means of summarizing and reporting large amounts of data. It is important to consider both the type and the distribution of the data before applying descriptive statistics.

The most common descriptive measure used is the mean, or the average. The mean can be noted by the Greek letter, μ. To calculate the mean, all of the values for all of the individuals in the data set are added and then the sum is divided by the total number of individuals in the sample.

$$\mu = \frac{\Sigma\, x_i}{n}$$

where μ = mean, Σ = sum of, x_i = individual value, n = sample size.

The median is the middle value when the data are arranged from the lowest value to the highest value. To determine the median, the data are arranged in ascending order. If the total sample size is an odd number, then the median is the number in the middle. If the total sample size is an even number, then the median is the average of the two middle numbers.

The mode is the value that occurs most frequently in the data set. Data sets can be unimodal, with only one mode, or multimodal with more than one mode. Figures 5-1, 5-2, and 5-3 are all examples of unimodal distributions, and Figure 5-4 is an example of a bimodal distribution.

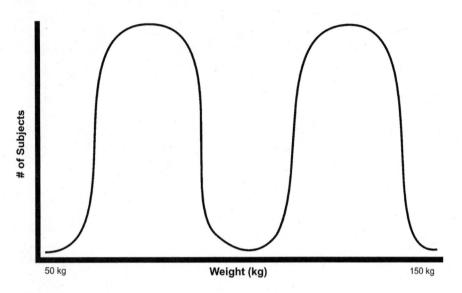

Figure 5-4. Bimodal distribution.

EXAMPLE 5-1

An investigator enrolls 10 boys ages 10 through 11 years in a study to investigate the effect of inhaled beclomethasone on growth rate. Table 5-3 lists the individual heights of the boys as well as mean height, median height, and mode for the group of boys.

To calculate the mean height of the boys in the sample, add all of the individual heights and divide the sum by the total number of children.

$$\mu \text{ height} = \frac{\Sigma x_i}{n} = \frac{52 + 53 + 53 + 53 + 54 + 55 + 56 + 57 + 58 + 59}{10}$$

$$= 55 \text{ inches}$$

TABLE 5-3. Height Distribution for a Sample of 10 Boys Ages 10-11

Subject	Height (inches)	Subject	Height (inches)
1	52	8	57
2	53	9	58
3	53	10	59
4	53	Mean	55
5	54	Median	54.5
6	55	Mode	53
7	56		

The median is the value in the middle of the sample when the data are arranged from lowest to highest. In this example, there is an even number of individuals in the sample; therefore, the median is obtained by taking the average of the two middle numbers. In this example, the median is calculated by averaging 54 and 55 inches for a median height of 54.5 inches.

The mode is the value that occurs most frequently in the sample. In this example, 53 inches is that value. It occurs 3 times in a sample of 10 individuals.

Measures of Dispersion

Several measures of dispersion are used to describe the variability in a given sample. These measures give an overview of how data are spread, or dispersed, in a sample.

The extremes are commonly used to describe the dispersion of a sample. The extremes are merely the lowest and the highest values in the data set. The range is also representative of the spread of the data set. The range is calculated by subtracting the lowest value from the highest value.

Percentiles are also useful in describing data. Percentiles indicate the percentage of individuals who have values equal to or below a given value. Some data are best reported in percentiles. Examples of variables consistently reported in percentiles are pediatric height and weight and standardized test scores. If a student receives a score of 93 on an examination and this places the student in the 90th percentile, then 90% of the students who took the same test scored equal to or lower than 93. The median represents the 50th percentile. If the median score on an examination is reported as 78, then 50% of students taking the test scored equal to or below 78.

The variance provides information about how individuals differ within the sample. The larger the variance, the more variability in the sample. The variance is calculated as follows:

$$S^2 = \frac{\Sigma(x_i - \mu)^2}{n - 1}$$

where S^2 = variance, Σ = sum of, x_i = individual value, μ = mean, n = sample size.

The standard deviation (SD) gives information about the variability of individuals around the mean. The larger the standard deviation, the more variability there is in the sample. In a normal distribution, some assumptions regarding the area under the curve can be made. As noted in Figure 5-5, 68% of individuals will fall between -1 and $+1$ SD, 95% of individuals will fall between -2 and $+2$ SD, and 99% of subjects will fall between -3 and $+3$ SD. The standard deviation is related to the variance. The standard deviation is the square root of the variance and can be calculated as follows:

$$SD = \sqrt{\text{variance}}$$

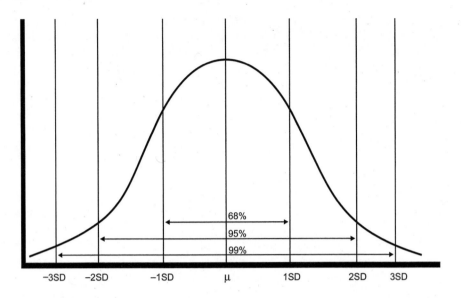

Figure 5-5. Area under the curve for a normal distribution.

or

$$SD = \sqrt{\frac{\Sigma(x_i - \mu)^2}{n - 1}}$$

The normal distribution of large samples (greater than 30 subjects) can be transformed into another distribution, called the z-distribution, which is similar to the standard normal distribution in that the area under both curves is equal to 1. In a z-distribution, the z-value on the x-axis represents how far an individual value is from the mean in units of standard deviation. Therefore, a z-value of 1 is equivalent to 1 standard deviation above the mean, and a z-value of −1 is equivalent to 1 standard deviation below the mean. The z-distribution is a probability curve. For example, Figure 5-6 shows that the probability of a value falling in a z-range of 1 to 2 is 13% (area under curve = 0.1358).

Small sample sizes (less than 30 subjects) are described using the t-distribution. Like the z-distribution, the t-distribution looks like a bell-shaped curve, is symmetrical, and contains an area under the curve that is equivalent to 1. The difference between the z- and t-distribution is the spread of the curve. The t-distribution is broader and flatter due to the smaller sample size. As shown in Figure 5-7, the smaller the sample size, the flatter and broader the t-distribution. As the sample size increases, the t-distribution more resembles the z-distribution.

The standard error (SE) is similar to the standard deviation. Whereas the standard deviation provides information about how individuals differ from the mean, the standard error provides information about the certainty of the mean itself. The distribution of the standard error is similar to the distribution of the standard deviation. The standard error can be calculated as follows:

$$SE = SD/\sqrt{n}$$

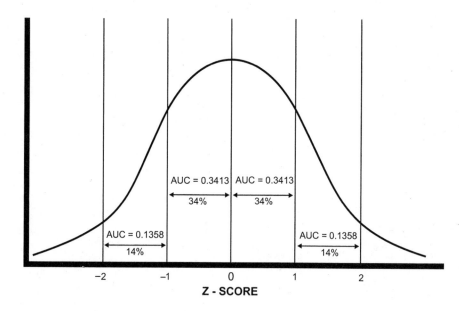

Figure 5-6. Area under the curve (AUC) for a *z*-distribution.

The standard error is interpreted much like the SD in that, the larger the standard error, the more uncertain the sample mean.

Confidence intervals (CI) are used to express the degree of confidence in an estimate. The confidence intervals can be calculated for any given estimate obtained from a sample. The confidence intervals denote the range of possible

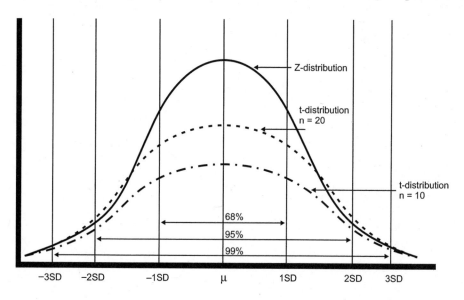

Figure 5-7. Effect of sample size on distribution.

values the estimate may assume, with a certain degree of assurance. For example, if the average low-density lipoprotein (LDL) for a group of subjects is 180 mg/dL and the 95% confidence intervals are (160, 200), then the investigators are 95% confident that the true mean LDL for the sample falls between 160 mg/dL and 200 mg/dL. Or, if a study is conducted 100 times, then 95 times out of 100 the mean LDL will fall between 160 mg/dL and 200 mg/dL. Remember that the mean obtained in any sample or study is an estimate. The 95% confidence intervals give information about the reliability of that estimate. The 95% confidence intervals of a mean can be calculated as follows:

$$95\% \text{ CI}_\mu = \mu \pm (2 \times \text{SE})$$

The confidence intervals can be calculated at various degrees of assurance. For example, it is possible to calculate the 90% confidence intervals or the 99% confidence intervals. The 99% confidence intervals would be interpreted to mean that there is 99% assurance that the estimate lies within the bounds of the confidence intervals. The most commonly reported confidence intervals are 95%. The confidence intervals are an important indicator of the reliability of the estimate. The narrower the confidence intervals, the more reliable is the estimate. For example, a mean age of 50 and a corresponding 95% confidence interval of (45, 55) is a more reliable estimate than a mean age of 50 in which the corresponding 95% confidence intervals is (30, 70). Confidence intervals also indicate the statistical significance of the results, which is discussed in detail later in this chapter.

EXAMPLE 5-2

Twelve subjects newly diagnosed with mild to moderate depression are enrolled into a clinical trial to evaluate the efficacy of St. John's Wort versus placebo for the treatment of depression. The individual ages of the individuals as well as the mean, median, range, extremes, variance, standard deviation, standard error, and 95% confidence intervals for each group are displayed in Table 5-4.

The mean ages of each group can be calculated as follows:

$$\mu \text{ age}_{\text{St. John's Wort group}} = \frac{\Sigma_i}{n} = \frac{36 + 21 + 24 + 20 + 30 + 25}{6} = 26$$

$$\mu \text{ age}_{\text{placebo group}} = \frac{\Sigma_i}{n} = \frac{35 + 46 + 38 + 44 + 36 + 45}{6} = 40.7$$

The median ages of each group are determined by arranging the ages in ascending order from the lowest age to the highest. Because the sample size is an even number, 6, the median age is obtained by averaging the two middle observations (observation $3 + 4$):

$$\text{ages in ascending order}_{\text{St. John's Wort}} = 20, 21, 24, 25, 30, 36$$

$$\text{median age}_{\text{St. John's Wort}} = \frac{24 + 25}{2} = 24.5$$

TABLE 5-4. **Data from a Study Comparing St. John's Wort Versus Placebo for Depression**

Observation	St. John's Wort Group Age (years)	Placebo Group Age (years)
1	36	35
2	21	46
3	24	38
4	20	44
5	30	36
6	25	45
Mean	26	40.7
Median	24.5	41
Range	16	11
Extremes	20, 36	35, 46
Variance	36.4	23.9
Standard deviation	6	4.9
Standard error	2.5	2
95% confidence intervals	(21, 31)	(36.7, 44.7)

$$\text{ages in ascending order}_{placebo} = 35, 36, 38, 44, 45, 46$$

$$\text{median age}_{placebo} = \frac{38 + 44}{2} = 41$$

The extremes are merely the lowest and the highest ages in each group. The range is obtained by subtracting the extremes in each group:

$$\text{Range}_{St. John's Wort} = 36 - 20 = 16$$
$$\text{Range}_{placebo} = 46 - 35 = 11$$

The variance and standard deviation for the St. John's Wort group and the placebo group are 182, 13.5 and 119.34, 10.9, respectively. They are calculated as follows:

$$\text{variance} = S^2 = \frac{\Sigma(x_i - \mu)^2}{n - 1}$$

$$SD = \sqrt{\text{variance}}$$

St. John's Wort group:

$$variance = \frac{(36-26)^2 + (21-26)^2 + (24-26)^2 + (20-26)^2 + (30-26)^2 + (25+26)^2}{6-1}$$

$$variance = 100 + 25 + 4 + 36 + 16 + 1 = \frac{182}{5} = 36.4$$

$$SD = \sqrt{36.4}$$
$$SD = 6.0$$

Placebo group:

$$variance = \frac{(35-40.7)^2 + (46-40.7)^2 + (38-40.7)^2 + (44-40.7)^2 + (36-40.7)^2 + (45+40.7)^2}{6-1}$$

$$variance = 32.49 + 28.09 + 7.29 + 10.89 + 22.09 + 18.49 = \frac{119.34}{5} = 23.9$$

$$SD = \sqrt{23.9}$$
$$SD = 4.9$$

Note that the variance and the standard deviation in the St. John's Wort group are slightly larger than the variance and the standard deviation in the placebo group. This result means that there is slightly more variability in age in the St. John's Wort group than in the placebo group.

The standard error for each group is calculated as follows:

$$SE_{SJW} = 6.0/\sqrt{6}$$
$$SE_{SJW} = 2.5$$
$$SE_{placebo} = 4.9/\sqrt{6}$$
$$SE_{placebo} = 2.0$$

As seen with the standard deviation, the standard error shows that there is more variability in age in the St. John's Wort group as compared with the placebo group.

The 95% confidence intervals can be calculated as follows:

$$95\% \ CI_{St. John's Wort} = 26 \pm 2(2.5) = (21, 31)$$

This finding can be interpreted to mean that there is 95% assurance that the true mean age for the St. John's Wort group lies between 21 years and 31 years or, if the study is conducted 100 times, then 95 times out of 100, the mean age will lie between 21 years and 31 years.

$$95\% \ CI_{placebo} = 40.7 \pm 2(2) = (36.7, 44.7)$$

There is 95% assurance that the true mean age for the placebo group lies between 36.7 years and 44.7 years or, if the study is conducted 100 times, then 95 times out of 100, the mean age will lie between 36.7 years and 44.7 years.

Application of Descriptive Measures

The type, dispersion, and distribution of data all should be considered before applying descriptive statistics. As mentioned previously, when data assume a normal distribution, the majority of values are clustered around the mean, or the center of the bell-shaped curve. In a normal distribution, the mean, median, and mode are equal. Therefore, any measure of central tendency will adequately describe a normally distributed data set. The mean and standard deviation are most commonly used to describe data sets that are normally distributed.

If the data assume a skewed distribution, however, then the mean and the median are not equal. In a skewed distribution, the mean is not located in the center of the curve. Therefore, the mean does not adequately describe the middle, or center, of a skewed distribution. In a skewed distribution, the median indicates the center of the distribution. Therefore, in a skewed distribution, the median and either the range or the extremes provide a much better description of the data set than the mean and the standard deviation. Percentiles can be used to describe both normally distributed and skewed data sets.

Inferential Methods

Once the data are collected, they are analyzed to determine any clinically relevant or statistically significant findings. Many statistical analyses can be used to analyze data. The most appropriate statistical test is determined by many factors. The data is statistically analyzed to test the null hypothesis. The null hypotheses are determined *à priori*, or before the study is actually conducted and the data are collected. Based on the results obtained in the sample studied, inferential methods are used to make inferences about populations.

Null Hypothesis

The null hypothesis (H_0) is a mathematical statement of equality stated before collecting or analyzing data. Typically, many null hypotheses are stated and tested in any given study. When comparing two groups, the null hypothesis is a mathematical statement that the groups are equal. If, for example, an investigator is interested in comparing lisinopril versus placebo for the treatment of hypertension, then one null hypothesis may be—

H_0: mean blood pressure at the end of study in the lisinopril group = mean blood pressure at the end of the study in the placebo group.

Once the null hypothesis has been stated and the data collected, the data are statistically analyzed and a p-value is calculated. Based on the calculated p-value, the null hypothesis will be either rejected or accepted. If there is no statistical difference between the two groups, then the null hypothesis will be accepted. Likewise, if there is a statistical difference between the two groups, then the null hypothesis will be rejected.

Statistical significance is determined solely by the calculated p-value, which is the probability that the result observed in the sample was due to chance. In a two-sample test, the p-value is the probability that the difference observed between the two groups was due to chance. A p-value of 0.05 indicates a 5% probability that the difference observed between the two groups was due to chance. A result corresponding to a p-value less than or equal to 0.05 is considered to be statistically significant and leads to rejection of the null hypothesis. In contrast, a p-value greater than 0.05 leads to acceptance of the null hypothesis.

It is important to note some limitations of the p-value. First, p-values are sensitive to sample size. The larger the sample size, the smaller the p-value. It is easier to achieve a statistically significant result with large samples than with small samples. Second, p-values are sensitive to the magnitude of the difference observed between two groups. Therefore, it is possible that very small differences observed between two groups in large samples will be statistically significant, but large differences observed between two groups in small samples will not be statistically significant. For these reasons, confidence intervals may sometimes provide more information than p-values. As noted previously, the CI provides information about both the statistical significance of the results and the reliability or the stability of the results.

Choosing the Appropriate Statistical Analysis

Many statistical tests are available to analyze data. In this book, a few of the most common tests are discussed. Numerous factors must be considered before determining which statistical test is most appropriate to analyze a particular data set. Appendix I displays the process for determining the most appropriate statistical test to use for a particular data set. The first consideration is whether the data are discrete or continuous. If the data are continuous, then the distribution of the data should be determined. Are the data normally distributed or skewed? If the data are discrete, then the expected counts should be calculated for each cell. Other general considerations include the number of groups in the study and whether the data are paired or unpaired. These considerations are discussed later in this chapter.

Statistical Analysis of Continuous Data

When data are identified to be continuous, it is important to identify whether the distribution is normally distributed or skewed. Null hypotheses tested in skewed distributions are different from null hypotheses tested in normal distributions. The statistical methods used to test the null hypotheses are different, depending on the distribution of data.

Statistical Analysis of Unpaired, Normally Distributed, Continuous Data

Unpaired continuous data that are normally distributed can be statistically analyzed using the t-test. When comparing two independent samples using the t-test, the null hypothesis states that the means of the two groups are equal. Figure 5-8 displays weight distributions for two groups in a study. These weights are normally

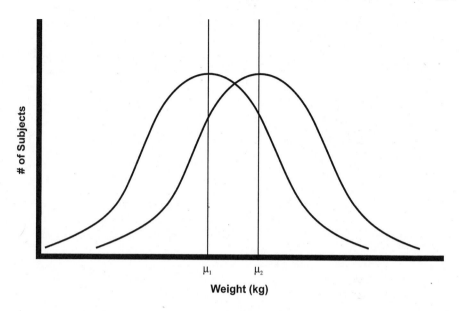

Figure 5-8. H_0: μ weight$_1$ = weight$_2$.

distributed in both groups, but the mean weights for each group are slightly different. The null hypothesis is that the mean weights for groups 1 and 2 are equal. The
statistical analysis will determine whether the mean weights for groups 1 and 2 are
statistically different.

Instructions to using the t-test for two independent samples are as follows:

1. State the null hypothesis to be tested via the t-test.

2. Calculate the means and variances for each group.

3. Calculate the pooled variance:

$$S_p^2 = \frac{(n_1 - 1)s_1^2 + (n_2 - 1)s_2^2}{n_1 + n_2 - 2}$$

where S_p^2 = pooled variance, n_1 = sample size group 1, s_1^2 = variance
group 1, n_2 = sample size group 2, s_2^2 = variance group 2

4. Calculate the t-value for the sample:

$$t = \frac{\mu_1 - \mu_2}{SE\,(\mu_1 - \mu_2)}$$

where $SE\,(\mu_1 - \mu_2) = S_p^2\sqrt{\dfrac{1}{n_1} + \dfrac{1}{n_2}}$

5. Use a t-value distribution table (see Appendix II) to determine the critical value of t. The critical value of t is the value of t required to reject the null hypothesis. The critical value of t changes, depending on the sample size. To use the t table, the degrees of freedom for the sample must be calculated. The degrees of freedom are related to the sample size and are calculated as follows:

$$df = n_1 + n_2 - 2$$

Appendix II is an abbreviated table of critical values of t required to reject the null hypothesis. A complete t-table would list all of the degrees of freedom from 1 through infinity.

Also listed in Appendix II are the critical t-values required to reject the null hypothesis for p-values 0.05, 0.01, and 0.001. As noted, a p-value $= 0.05$ is most commonly used to reject the null hypothesis. If the calculated t-value falls within the range of positive and negative critical values of t obtained from the table, then the null hypothesis is accepted. If the calculated t-value from the sample falls in either of the tails, then the null hypothesis is rejected. In other words, if the calculated t-value from the sample is less than the negative critical value of t or greater than the positive critical value of t, then the null hypothesis is rejected.

6. Interpret and report the results of the analysis:

The 95% CI for the difference between the two means can be calculated as follows:

$$95\% \text{ CI} = (\mu_1 - \mu_2) \pm t_{df}\sqrt{s_p^2\left(\frac{1}{n_1} + \frac{1}{n_2}\right)}$$

As noted previously, the larger the sample size, the narrower the confidence intervals.

EXAMPLE 5-3

Subjects with mild to moderate hypertension are enrolled in a study and randomly assigned to drug A or drug B for the treatment of hypertension. Diastolic blood pressure (DBP) is measured at baseline, and every 4 weeks for 6 months. Table 5-5 displays the DBP measurements for each subject at baseline and at 6 months. Using Appendix I, the t-test is determined to be the most appropriate test for analyzing the data because the study compares two groups for which the data are unpaired, continuous, and normally distributed.

The data in Table 5-5 can be statistically analyzed using the t-test as follows:

1. State the null hypothesis to be tested via the t-test.

H_0: mean DBP at 6 months$_{\text{drug A}}$ = mean DBP at 6 months$_{\text{drug B}}$

or

H_0: mean DBP at 6 months$_{\text{drug A}}$ − mean DBP at 6 months$_{\text{drug B}}$ = 0

TABLE 5-5. **Diastolic Blood Pressure Measurements at Baseline and 6 Months in 20**

	Drug A			Drug B		
Sub-ject	DBP at Baseline (mm Hg)	DBP at 6 months (mm Hg)	DBP Difference 6 months – Baseline (mm Hg)	DBP at Baseline (mm Hg)	DBP at 6 months (mm Hg)	DBP Difference 6 months – Base-line (mm Hg)
1	85	80	$85 - 80 = 5$	86	82	$86 - 82 = 4$
2	90	88	$90 - 88 = 2$	90	83	$90 - 83 = 7$
3	88	81	$88 - 81 = 7$	90	82	$90 - 82 = 8$
4	89	92	$89 - 92 = -3$	88	85	$88 - 85 = 3$
5	95	90	$95 - 90 = 5$	93	86	$93 - 86 = 7$
6	92	95	$92 - 95 = -3$	95	90	$95 - 90 = 5$
7	86	84	$86 - 84 = 2$	88	81	$88 - 81 = 7$
8	85	81	$85 - 81 = 4$	85	83	$85 - 83 = 2$
9	92	85	$92 - 85 = 7$	91	89	$91 - 89 = 2$
10	100	93	$100 - 93 = 7$	86	81	$86 - 81 = 5$
Σ	902	869	33	892	842	50
Group mean	90.2	86.9	3.3	89.2	84.2	5

Note: DBP 5 diastolic blood pressure

2. Calculate the means and variances for each group.

$$\text{mean DBP}_{\text{drug A}} = \frac{80 + 88 + 81 + 92 + 90 + 95 + 84 + 81 + 85 + 93}{10}$$

$$= 86.9 \text{ mm Hg}$$

$$\text{mean DBP}_{\text{drug B}} = \frac{82 + 83 + 82 + 85 + 86 + 90 + 81 + 83 + 89 + 81}{10}$$

$$= 84.2 \text{ mm Hg}$$

$$S_1^2 = \frac{\begin{array}{l}(80 - 86.9)^2 + (88 - 86.9)^2 + (81 - 86.9)^2 + (92 - 86.9)^2 \\ + (90 - 86.9)^2 + (95 - 86.9)^2 + (84 - 86.9)^2 + (81 - 86.9)^2 \\ + (85 - 86.9)^2 + (93 - 86.9)^2\end{array}}{10 - 1}$$

$S_1^2 = 29.88$

$$S_2^2 = \frac{\begin{array}{c}(82 - 84.2)^2 + (83 - 84.2)^2 + (82 - 84.2)^2 + (85 - 84.2)^2 \\ + (86 - 84.2)^2 + (90 - 84.2)^2 + (81 - 84.2)^2 + (83 - 84.2)^2 \\ + (89 - 84.2)^2 + (81 - 84.2)^2\end{array}}{10 - 1}$$

$S_2^2 = 10.4$

3. Calculate the pooled variance.

$$S_p^2 = \frac{(n_1 - 1)s_1^2 + (n_2 - 1)s_2^2}{n_1 + n_2 - 2}$$

where S_p^2 = pooled variance, n_1 = sample size group 1, s_1^2 = variance group 1, n_2 = sample size group 2, s_2^2 = variance group 2

$$S_p^2 = \frac{(10 - 1)\,29.88 + (10 - 1)\,10.4}{10 + 10 - 2}$$

$$S_p^2 = 20.14$$

4. Calculate the t-value.

$$t = \frac{\mu_1 - \mu_2}{SE\,(\mu_1 - \mu_2)}$$

where $SE\,(\mu_1 - \mu_2) = S_p^2\sqrt{\dfrac{1}{n_1} + \dfrac{1}{n_2}}$

$$t = \frac{86.9 - 84.2}{20.14\sqrt{\dfrac{1}{10} + \dfrac{1}{10}}}$$

$$t = 0.2997$$

5. Use a t-value distribution table (see Appendix II) to determine the critical value of t. The degrees of freedom for the t-test are as follows:

$$df = n_1 + n_2 - 2$$

Figure 5-9 shows that for df = 18, the critical t-value required to reject the null hypothesis is 2.101. Therefore, any calculated t-value greater than or equal to 2.101 or less than −2.101 will lead to rejection of the null hypothesis. If the calculated t-value falls within the range from −2.101 to 2.101, then the null hypothesis is accepted. In this example, the calculated value of t is equal to 0.2997, and this value falls within the range of −2.101 and 2.101; therefore, the null hypothesis is accepted.

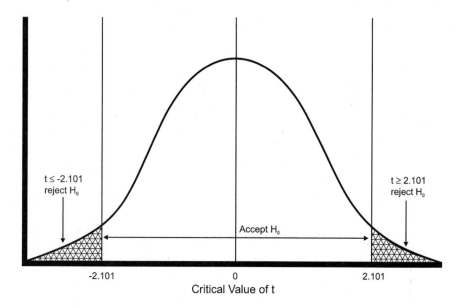

t ≤ -2.101
reject H₀

t ≥ 2.101
reject H₀

Accept H₀

-2.101   0   2.101
Critical Value of t

Figure 5-9. Critical values of t for example 5-3.

6. Interpret and report the results of the analysis:
The mean DBP in the drug A group at 6 months is not statistically different
from the mean DBP at 6 months in the drug B group.

Statistical Analysis of Paired, Normally Distributed, Continuous Data

Paired continuous data that are normally distributed can be statistically analyzed
using the paired t-test. When comparing two independent samples using the
paired t-test, the null hypothesis states that the mean differences between the two
groups is equal. The data collected and shown in Table 5-5 could be analyzed
using the paired t-test. Although the t-test uses only one measurement per subject
and thus compares the mean DBP in each group at 6 months, the paired t-test uses
two measurements per subject and thus compares the mean differences in DBP in
each group. The mean differences in DBP for each group are also displayed in
Table 5-5. To calculate the mean difference for each group, first calculate the
difference for each subject by subtracting the DBP at 6 months from the DBP at
baseline. Then, simply add up all of the individual differences and divide by the
sample size. The mean differences for each group in this example are calculated as
follows:

$$\text{mean difference group}_A = \frac{\begin{array}{c}(85 - 80) + (90 - 88) + (88 - 81) + (89 - 92) \\ + (95 - 90) + (92 - 95) + (86 - 84) \\ + (85 - 81) + (92 - 85) + (100 - 93)\end{array}}{10} = 3.3$$

The mean DBP decreased by 3.3 mm Hg for group A.

$$\text{mean difference group}_B = \frac{\begin{array}{c}(86 - 82) + (90 - 83) + (90 - 82) + (88 - 85) \\ + (93 - 86) + (95 - 90) + (88 - 81) \\ + (85 - 83) + (91 - 89) + (86 - 81)\end{array}}{10} = 5.0$$

The mean DBP decreased by 5 mm Hg for group B.

The paired t-test is similar to the t-test. In this example, the null hypothesis states that the mean differences in DBP (baseline DBP − 6 month DBP) are the same for both groups. Next, the t-value is calculated and compared to the critical value of t required to reject the null hypothesis. If the null hypothesis is rejected, then the mean differences between the two groups are statistically different, and one therapy is more effective than the other. If the null hypothesis is not rejected, then the mean differences are not statistically different and the therapies are equal.

Statistical Analysis of Skewed Continuous Data

There are statistical tests designed specifically for continuous data that are skewed. These tests compare the medians of two groups. As noted previously, the mean does not adequately describe a skewed distribution, which is why it is not appropriate to use parametric tests on skewed data. Instead, nonparametric tests are used. The Wilcoxon Rank Sum or the Mann Whitney Test can be used for unpaired skewed data. The Wilcoxon Signed Rank test can be used for paired skewed data.

Whereas parametric analyses test the null hypothesis that the means of two groups are equal, nonparametric analyses test the null hypothesis that the medians of two groups are equal. Suppose a study is conducted to evaluate a steroid inhaler versus an oral steroid for the treatment of asthma. Forced expiratory volume (FEV) is measured at baseline and every 2 weeks for 4 months. The FEV distribution in both groups is skewed, so a nonparametric test will be used. Figure 5-10 shows that the null hypothesis states that the median FEV at 4 months for the steroid inhaler group is equal to the median FEV at 4 months for the oral steroid group. A paired analysis would test the null hypothesis that the median differences in FEV (FEV at 4 months 2 FEV at baseline) are equal for both groups.

Statistical Analysis of Discrete Data

Certain statistical tests are designed specifically for the purpose of analyzing discrete data. The Chi-Square Test and the Fisher's Exact Test are two statistical tests that are commonly used to analyze discrete data. The Chi-Square test is used to analyze large samples, and the Fisher's Exact Test is used to analyze small samples. The null hypotheses for both of these tests are the same. Because these tests analyze discrete data, the null hypotheses are based on proportions. Therefore, when comparing discrete data in two independent groups, the null hypothesis states that

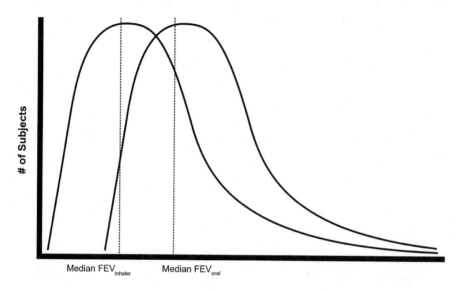

Figure 5-10. H_0: median $FEV_{inhaled\ steroid}$ = median $FEV_{oral\ steroid}$.

the proportions of a characteristic or event in the two groups are equal.
Instructions to use the Chi-Square Test for two independent samples are as
follows:

1. State the null hypothesis to be tested via the Chi-Square Test.

2. Plot the observed frequencies in a 2 × 2 contingency table. Each subject
will fit into only one cell of the contingency table. Table 5-6 displays the
observed frequencies.

3. Based on the observed frequencies in each cell, calculate the corresponding
expected frequency for each cell. The expected frequencies can be calculated
by multiplying the row total times the column total and then dividing the

TABLE 5-6. **Observed Frequencies**

		Outcome		Total
		Yes	No	
EXPOSURE	Yes	A	B	A + B
	No	C	D	C + D
		A + C	B + D	A + B + C + D

TABLE 5-7. Formulas for Calculating Expected Frequencies

		Outcome		Total
		Yes	No	
EXPOSURE	Yes	$\dfrac{(A + B)(A + C)}{n}$	$\dfrac{(A + B)(B + D)}{n}$	A + B
	No	$\dfrac{(C + D)(A + C)}{n}$	$\dfrac{(C + D)(B + D)}{n}$	C + D
		A + C	B + D	A + B + C + D

result by the total sample size. The calculations for the expected frequencies are shown in Table 5-7.

4. Count the number of expected cells with frequencies ≤ 5. If more than 25% of the expected cells contain frequencies ≤ 5, then the Fisher's Exact Test must be used to analyze the data. If 25% or fewer of the expected cells contain frequencies ≤ 5, then the Chi-Square Test can be used to analyze the data. This means, in a 2×2 contingency table, only one of the four expected cells can have a frequency of 5 or less. If more than one expected cell in a 2×2 contingency table has a frequency ≤ 5, then the Fisher's Exact Test must be used instead.

5. Calculate a Chi-Square critical value. The Chi-Square critical value is calculated as follows:

$$\text{Chi-Square} = \Sigma \left\{ \frac{(O - E)^2}{E} \right\}$$

where Σ = sum of, O = observed value, and E = expected value

6. Use a Chi-Square distribution table (see Appendix III) to determine the critical X^2 value required to reject the null hypothesis for the degrees of freedom calculated from the sample. The X^2 critical values required to reject the null hypothesis are listed in Appendix II for p-values of 0.05, 0.01, and 0.001. The degrees of freedom in a Chi-Square Test are calculated as follows:

$$\text{degrees of freedom} = (R - 1)(C - 1)$$

where df = degrees of freedom, R = number of rows, and
C = number of columns

If the calculated X^2-value from the sample is greater than or equal to the X^2 critical value obtained from the table, then the null hypothesis is rejected. If the calculated X^2-value from the sample is less than the X^2 critical value, then the null hypothesis is accepted. In a 2×2 contingency table, the degrees of freedom equal 1, and the critical X^2 required to reject the null hypothesis is equal to 3.84. Therefore, any calculated X^2-value greater than or equal to 3.84 will lead to rejection of the null hypothesis. A calculated X^2-value less than 3.84 will lead to acceptance of the null hypothesis.

7. Interpret and report the results of the analysis.

EXAMPLE 5-4

An investigator enrolls 123 subjects into a study evaluating St. John's Wort versus placebo for the treatment of depression. The gender distributions for the two groups are slightly different. Twenty-six of the 63 subjects assigned to the St. John's Wort are male, and 21 of the 60 subjects assigned to the placebo group are male. The investigator would like to statistically compare the two groups to determine whether the gender distributions are statistically different. Appendix I can be used to determine the most appropriate test to analyze the data. Because gender is a discrete, unpaired variable and the investigator is comparing two groups, the Chi-Square Test is appropriate to analyze the data.

The Chi-Square test can be applied to Example 5-4 as follows:

1. State the null hypothesis.

$$H_0: \text{Proportion of males}_{\text{St. John's Wort}} = \text{Proportion of males}_{\text{placebo}}$$

The Chi-Square Test will be used to test the hypothesis that the proportion of males is equal in the two groups. The proportion of males in each group is easily calculated. For the St. John's Wort group, the proportion of males is 26/63, or 41%, whereas the proportion of males in the placebo group is 21/60, or 35%. Statistical analysis of these proportions will determine if this gender difference observed between the 2 groups is statistically significant. If the proportion of males in the two groups is statistically different, then the null hypothesis will be rejected.

2. Plot the observed frequencies in a 2×2 contingency table. The observed frequencies are plotted in Table 5-8.

TABLE 5-8. Observed Gender Frequencies in a Study

	Male	Female	Total
ST. JOHN'S WORT	26	37	63
PLACEBO	21	39	60
	47	76	123

TABLE 5-9. **Expected Gender Frequencies in a Study**

	Male	*Female*	*Total*
ST. JOHN'S WORT	$\dfrac{(26 + 37)(26 + 21)}{123} = 24$	$\dfrac{(26 + 37)(37 + 39)}{123} = 39$	63
PLACEBO	$\dfrac{(21 + 39)(26 + 21)}{123} = 23$	$\dfrac{(21 + 39)(37 + 39)}{123} = 37$	60
	47	76	123

3. Calculate the corresponding expected frequency for each cell. The expected frequencies are shown in Table 5-9.

4. Count the number of expected cells with frequencies equal to or less than 5. Because none of the expected frequencies in this example is less than or equal to 5, it is appropriate to use the Chi-Square Test to analyze the data.

5. Calculate a Chi-Square value.

$$X^2 = \Sigma \left\{ \frac{(O - E)^2}{E} \right\}$$

$$X^2 = \frac{(26 - 24)^2}{24} + \frac{(37 - 39)^2}{39} + \frac{(21 - 23)^2}{23} + \frac{(39 - 37)^2}{37}$$

$$X^2 = 0.5513$$

6. Use a Chi-Square distribution table (see Appendix III) to determine the critical X^2-value required to reject the null hypothesis for the degrees of freedom calculated from the sample. The calculated X^2-value is 0.5513, with degrees of freedom = $(R - 1)(C - 1)$; degrees of freedom = $(2 - 1)$ $(2 - 1) = 1$. The X^2 critical value required to reject the null hypothesis at $p = 0.05$ for degrees of freedom = 1 is 3.84. Figure 5-11 shows that because the calculated X^2 value (0.5513) is less than the X^2 critical value (3.84), the null hypothesis is accepted.

7. Interpret and report the results of the analysis:
The proportion of males in the St. John's Wort group is not statistically different from the proportion of males in the placebo group.

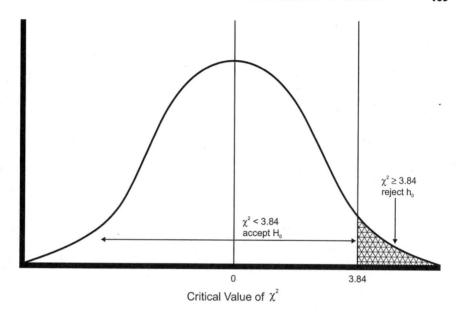

$\chi^2 \geq 3.84$
reject h_0

$\chi^2 < 3.84$
accept H_0

0   3.84

Critical Value of χ^2

Figure 5-11. Critical values of χ^2 for example 5-4.

Interpretation of Results

There are other considerations when interpreting the results of a study. Both the sample size and the power of the study should be considered. As noted, the sample size, which is determined during the design phase of the study, influences the likelihood of achieving a statistically significant result. The preferred levels of both α (type I error rate) and β (type II error rate) are included in the sample size calculation. Investigators typically set the α at 0.05 and the β at 0.2.

The other determinant of sample size is the magnitude of the difference the investigator wishes to detect between the two groups. The magnitude of the difference is typically guided by prior study results on the same or similar drugs. The smaller the difference the investigator wishes to detect between two groups, the larger the sample size needed. Conversely, gross differences between groups require smaller sample sizes. Consider a study in which an investigator is designing a study to compare drug A to a placebo for weight loss in obese subjects. The sample size required to detect a difference of 5 pounds between two groups will be much larger than the sample size required to detect a difference of 20 pounds between two groups. Sometimes, a study does not show a statistically significant result solely because the sample size was inadequate. The results, however, are highly suggestive of an important and useful trend. Conversely, a study with a very large sample size can show statistical significance despite a very small difference observed between two groups.

Power refers to the strength or ability of a study to detect a given difference between groups. As stated previously, the difference the investigator wishes to detect between two groups is decided in the design phase of the study and included in the sample size calculation. Sample size is related to power. As the sample size increases, so does the power of the study. The power is also influenced by the magnitude of the difference observed between two groups. As the magnitude increases, the power increases. Power can be calculated by $1-\beta$. Because β is usually set at 20%, investigators typically design studies with a goal of achieving at least 80% power.

Regardless of the statistical results of the study, it is imperative to determine the clinical relevance of the actual study results. Many studies show statistically significant results, but the results are not clinically relevant. *Clinical relevance* refers to the utility of the results in actual practice. A finding that is clinically relevant, for example, will result in one drug being used over another. For example, a comparison of two diet suppressants may yield results such that group A has a mean weight loss of 3 pounds and group B has a mean weight loss of 5 pounds. This result may be statistically significant, but the actual results will not convince physicians to prescribe drug B over drug A.

Summary

When designing, conducting, and evaluating a study, many issues must be considered, especially with regard to describing and analyzing collected data. Descriptive measures can be used to provide a summary of the data, and inferential methods can be used to make inferences about the population based on the sample. When determining the relevance of the results of the study, considerations such as sample size and power should be taken into account. Smaller studies may never exhibit statistical significance or demonstrate adequate power, but they can provide important and valuable information. After evaluating the quality of the study design and analysis, the clinical relevance of the results must be considered. A large, well-designed study that shows a statistical difference between two drug therapies may have no clinical relevance in practice. Also important are p-values and statistical significance, but they should not determine the application of study results to clinical practice. If the difference observed between two drug therapies is not enough to convince practitioners to use one drug over another, then the statistical significance of the results is irrelevant. The quality of the study, the statistical results, and the clinical relevance of the results all should be considered when determining the utility of a particular study.

References

1. Rosner BA. *Fundamentals of Biostatistics.* 4th ed. Wadsworth Publishing Company; 1995.

2. Dawson-Saunders B, Trapp RG. *Basic and Clinical Biostatistics.* 2nd ed. Norwalk, Conn.: Appleton & Lange; 1994.

Study Questions

1. For each of the five variables listed here, indicate which type of data each represents. The choices are discrete and continuous.

   a. season
   b. HIV status
   c. Viral load
   d. CPK
   e. orthopnea

Questions 2 through 8 refer to data collected in a study evaluating an herbal medication versus a placebo for the treatment or rheumatoid arthritis (RA). Table 5-10 displays data collected during the study.

2. The variable, number of years diagnosed with RA, is a continuous variable measured in years. Explain how this variable can be transformed into a discrete variable.

3. For the continuous variable, number of years diagnosed with RA, calculate the following measures for both the herbal medication and the placebo groups:

   a. mean
   b. median

TABLE 5-10. **Data from a Study Comparing Herbal Medication Versus Placebo for Treatment of Rheumatoid Arthritis**

	Placebo Group			Herbal Group		
Obser-vation	Number of Years With RA	Degree of Pain at Baseline*	Degree of Pain at End of Study*	Number of Years With RA	Degree of Pain at Baseline*	Degree of Pain at End of Study*
1	5	4	4	4	3	3
2	7	4	5	6	2	3
3	6	3	2	5	4	5
4	9	3	4	7	2	2
5	12	5	5	7	3	2
6	8	3	5	5	2	3
7	10	2	3	9	2	2
8	11	4	5	8	3	2

Note: RA 5 rheumatoid arthritis.
*Scale: 1 through 5, with 1 being least pain and 5 being most pain.

   c. variance

   d. standard deviation

   e. standard error

   f. 95% confidence intervals of the mean

4. Which is the most appropriate statistical test to use in analyzing whether the variable, mean number of years diagnosed with RA, differs statistically between the placebo and the herbal medication groups?

5. Use the appropriate statistical test to analyze the data provided in Table 5-10 and determine if the mean number of years diagnosed with RA is equal in the two groups.

6. What type of variable is degree of pain?

7. Which statistical test is most appropriate to analyze the degree of pain in the two groups at the end of the study?

8. Which statistical test is most appropriate to analyze the degree of pain relief in the two groups?

9. A survey study of 500 men and 700 women was conducted to determine what percent of Americans used herbal medications in the past year. Twenty-five percent of men and 34% of women reported using an herbal medication in the past year. Using the appropriate statistical test, determine whether herbal medication use is statistically different for men compared with women.

Chapter 6

Risk Assessment

Risk measures are estimates that describe the amount of risk associated with a particular exposure in a sample population. Risk estimates can quantitatively describe the risk associated with a particular exposure and the development or prevention of disease, and they can quantify the association between the exposure to a particular drug and an adverse drug reaction.

Risk estimates are part of our daily lives. Measures of risk are communicated to patients via newspapers, television, and the Internet daily. Risk measures are communicated to practitioners via studies published in medical journals. These risk measures become important in the clinical decision-making process for both patients and practitioners.

It is important to have a clear understanding of risk measures to appropriately interpret and apply the estimates. Risk measures are difficult to use for many reasons, including the conflicting results obtained from different studies. For example, early observational studies have reported a positive association[1-3] between calcium channel blocker use and cancer, whereas more recent observational studies have reported a negative association.[4,5] When conflicting information pertaining to risk is published, it becomes difficult for both practitioners and patients to use risk estimates for clinical decision-making. A clear understanding of study design and the derivation of risk estimates allows practitioners to determine the most reliable risk estimates to use in the midst of conflicting results.

Additional confusion exists around the actual interpretation of the results of a study regarding risk estimates. Two readers may interpret, communicate, and use the results of a study very differently. Note, for example, the headlines that appeared on January 1, 1998, in two newspapers. Both newspapers reported the results of the same study on their front pages. The study assessed the risk of body weight and death. Interestingly, the two newspaper writers arrived at opposing interpretations of the study results, as evidenced by the titles of their stories. The headline in one newspaper read, "Adding Pounds as the Years Pass Increases Death Risk, Study Finds," whereas the headline in the second newspaper read, "Study Shows Obesity Poses Less of a Risk Than Thought." These two reporters read the same study, interpreted the results, and communicated conflicting summaries, leaving the reader to decipher the actual risks of weight gain. When we rely on others to summarize study results involving risk estimates, we are often faced with conflicting results, depending on the writer's skills and perspective. The more adept a pharmacist becomes in evaluating and interpreting risk estimates, the more effective he or she will be in helping patients to sort through the conflicting information they receive.

Prevalence and Incidence

A discussion of measures of risk should include a review of prevalence and incidence. *Prevalence* (P) is defined as the number of existing cases of disease (or any outcome, e.g., adverse drug reaction, drug use) in a population at a particular point in time.

$$P = \frac{\text{number of existing cases in a population}}{\text{total number of people in that population}}$$

Example 6-1

On January 1, 1999, college X had 3000 students enrolled. On January 1, 1999, 300 students at college X reported using an albuterol inhaler daily.

$$P = \frac{300}{3000} = 0.10, \text{ or } 10\%.$$

Therefore, on January 1, 1999, 10% of the students at college X used an albuterol inhaler daily. In other words, the prevalence of albuterol inhaler use on January 1, 1999, was 10%.

Medication use can often be used as a surrogate measure for prevalence of disease. A *surrogate measure* is an indirect measure of an outcome of interest. If access to data on disease status are unavailable, then an investigator may choose to use a surrogate measure, such as drug use, to represent presence or absence of disease. Sometimes, owing to time and expense limitations, it is not feasible to study the actual outcome of interest. In this example, a direct measurement of asthma prevalence would require obtaining and reviewing the medical records of all of the students at college X, which would be an arduous task. Instead, students were asked to report on the daily use of albuterol inhalers. In this scenario, albuterol use became a surrogate measure for prevalence of asthma. Although surrogate measures are more expedient and convenient than measuring actual outcomes, there are several limitations to their use. In this example, there were some major limitations in substituting albuterol use as a surrogate measure for asthma:

1. Not all asthmatics require albuterol daily.

2. Not all subjects who use albuterol have a diagnosis of asthma.

Another example of the use of surrogate measures is substituting blood pressure as an outcome in a study of the effectiveness of antihypertensive medications. Patients with high blood pressure take antihypertensive medications for the ultimate outcome of preventing stroke and myocardial infarction (MI); however, most studies evaluating antihypertensive medications use decreased blood pressure as the desirable endpoint or outcome, rather than measuring stroke and MI events. The time and expense involved in following patients for decades to determine the number of strokes and MIs precludes most investigators from designing such studies. Instead, the study design assumes that if the antihypertensive medication lowers blood pressure, then there will be a long-term benefit of decreased risk of stroke and MI.

Incidence (I) is defined as the number of new cases of disease that develop in a population at risk over a specified time period. Incidence is used to determine how often the disease is occurring. Incidence is typically described as either cumulative incidence (CI) or an incidence rate (IR). Cumulative incidence assumes that all of the subjects were followed for the entire study period. Cumulative incidence does not reflect study dropouts or losses to follow-up.

$$CI = \frac{\text{number of new cases disease during given time}}{\text{total population at risk}}$$

Example 6-2

Using college X in example 6-1, during the time frame of January 1, 1999, through December 31, 1999, 30 students started using albuterol.

$$CI = \frac{30}{3000 - 300} = 0.011, \text{ or } 1.1\% \text{ per year}$$

For the time period from January 1, 1999, through December 31, 1999, 1.1% of students at college X started using albuterol. The incidence of albuterol use in college X was 1.1% per year.

Note that the prevalence of albuterol use on January 1, 1999, is subtracted from the denominator. Incidence measures the risk of developing the disease or outcome of interest in a population at risk; therefore, any subjects who currently have the disease or outcome of interest at the onset of the study period are subtracted from the denominator. If a subject already has the disease, then the subject is not at risk for developing the disease and, therefore, cannot be included in the population at risk.

Incidence rate (IR), also referred to as *incidence density* (ID), is a more accurate means of measuring disease occurrence. Incidence rate takes into account the actual observation time of each subject during the study period, rather than assuming that all subjects were followed for the entire study period.

$$IR = \frac{\text{number of new cases}}{\text{total person-time of observation in population at risk}}$$

Example 6-3

Using the same college X study conducted from January 1, 1999, through December 31, 1999, assume that 12 students started using albuterol 3 months into the study, and 18 students started using albuterol 6 months into the study. Of the remaining students in the study, 300 drop out after 4 months, and 600 drop out after 8 months.

$$IR = \frac{30}{(12 \times 3 \text{ months}) + (18 \times 6 \text{ months}) + (300 \times 4 \text{ months}) + (600 \times 8 \text{ months}) + (1770 \times 12 \text{ months})}$$

$$IR = \frac{30}{27{,}384 \text{ person-months}}$$

$$= 0.0010955$$

$$= 0.11\% \text{ of students develop asthma per person-month}$$

To get the person-years equivalent, multiply 0.0010955 by 12 months per year, 0.013 students develop asthma per person-year.

$$IR = \frac{30}{2282} \text{ person-years} = 0.013$$

For every 100 person-years of observation, 1.3 students at college X develop asthma.

Notice the slight difference between the cumulative incidence of 1.1% and the incidence rate of 1.3%. Although in this example the cumulative incidence is less than the incidence rate, the cumulative incidence typically overestimates the occurrence of disease.

It is important to remember that a relationship exists between prevalence and incidence. In most situations, where incidence is constant and prevalence is low, prevalence is approximately equal to incidence multiplied by duration. For example, for a condition such as heart disease, with which people live a long time, the prevalence is high. For conditions such as colon cancer, of which people do not live long, the prevalence is low.

A tool used to calculate risk estimates is the *contingency table*. These tables are used to analyze discrete data. As discussed in Chapter 5, discrete data can take on a finite number of values. In a contingency table, each subject in the study is plotted once according to the presence or the absence of both exposure and outcome. Typically, outcome (e.g., development of disease, adverse drug reaction) is plotted downward, and exposure status is plotted across the table. A contingency table can have an infinite number of rows and columns but, for the purposes of this chapter, contingency tables will have 2 rows and 2 columns, referred to as a 2 × 2 table, as shown in Table 6-1:

TABLE 6-1. **2 × 2 Contingency Table**

| | | DISEASE/OUTCOME | | |
		Yes	No	Total
EXPOSURE	Yes	A	B	Total exposed
	No	C	D	Total unexposed
		Total with disease	Total without disease	n

Each subject gets counted in only **one** box.

Individuals in box **A** have been exposed and developed the disease.

Individuals in box **B** have been exposed but did **not** develop the disease.

Individuals in box **C** have **not** been exposed but still developed the disease.

Individuals in box **D** have **not** been exposed and did **not** develop the disease.

Note that if boxes **A** and **B** are added, the sum is total number of subjects in the study who were exposed. Adding boxes **C** and **D** yields the total number of subjects in the study who were **not** exposed. In the same regard, adding boxes **A** and **C** gives the total number of subjects who developed the disease. Adding boxes **B** and **D** provides the total number of subjects who did **not** develop the disease. Finally, the sum of boxes **A, B, C,** and **D** yields the total number of subjects in the study (sample size, or n).

Cumulative incidence can be obtained from a 2 × 2 table. Using Table 6-1, cumulative incidence is calculated for both the exposed and the unexposed groups as follows:

$$CI_{exposed} = \frac{A}{A + B}$$

$$CI_{unexposed} = \frac{C}{C + D}$$

Example 6-4

Using college X as an example, assume that 3000 students are enrolled. Three hundred students have asthma before starting the year. Of the 2700 remaining students, 1400 students live in the city and 1300 students live in the country. Of the students who live in the city, 200 develop asthma during the school year. Of the students who live in the country, 100 students develop asthma during the school year. In this example, living in the city becomes an exposure and is plotted against the outcome, development of asthma.

The cumulative incidence of asthma among college X students who live in the city and college X students who live in the country can be calculated using a 2 × 2

TABLE 6-2. 2 × 2 Contingency Table Comparing City Living Versus Country Living and the Development of Asthma

		ASTHMA		
		Yes	No	Total
LIVE IN	Yes	200	1200	1400
THE CITY	No	100	1200	1300
		300	2400	2700

contingency table. First, each student should be plotted according to exposure and outcome into the 2 × 2 contingency table. Remember, each student will fit into only one cell of the contingency table. Living in the city will be used as the exposure. Table 6-2 shows that students who live in the city and develop asthma are plotted in cell A, whereas students who live in the city and do not develop asthma are plotted in cell B. Students who do not live in the city and develop asthma are plotted in cell C, and students who do not live in the city and do not develop asthma are plotted in cell D.

First, to calculate the cumulative incidence of asthma in the exposed group (students who live in the city)—

$$CI_{exposed} = \frac{A}{A + B}$$

$$CI_{exposed} = \frac{200}{1400}$$

$$= 0.1428$$

$$= 14.28\% \text{ of students living in the city develop asthma per year}$$

Next, to calculate the cumulative incidence of asthma in the unexposed group (students who do **not** live in the city)—

$$CI_{unexposed} = \frac{C}{C + D}$$

$$CI_{unexposed} = \frac{100}{1300}$$

$$= 0.0769$$

$$= 7.69\% \text{ of students living in the country develop asthma per year}$$

Relative Risk

Once the incidence of an outcome or disease has been measured in both the exposed and the unexposed groups, it is useful to know the relationship between exposure and development of disease. Relative risk (RR) is the likelihood of developing the disease in the exposed group relative to the unexposed group; it is a measure of association between the exposure and the disease. It is important to remember that relative risk measures are *estimates*. They are risk estimates derived from a particular study population. The actual, or true, risk in the population at large may be greater or less than the risk estimate derived from the study sample. Relative risk is simply a ratio of the cumulative incidence in the exposed group over the cumulative incidence in the unexposed group and can be calculated as follows:

$$RR = \frac{CI_{exposed}}{CI_{unexposed}} = \frac{A/A + B}{C/C + D}$$

Relative risk can be estimated from a 2 × 2 contingency table. The null hypothesis in a comparison of two groups states that the proportion of subjects with the outcome of interest is equal in the exposed and the unexposed groups. In other words, the relative risk equals 1.

Relative risk can be used to measure the association between exposure and outcome in cohort studies and clinical trials. The relative risk is not used in the context of a case-control study, which is discussed later in this chapter. As noted in Table 6-3, a relative risk equal to 1 means there is no association between exposure and outcome. Essentially, a relative risk of 1 is, in fact, the null hypothesis. A relative risk less than 1 represents a decreased risk, or negative association, between exposure and outcome, also referred to as a *protective effect*. A relative risk greater than 1 represents an increased risk, or positive association, between exposure and outcome.

Example 6-5

The relative risk for developing asthma for college X students living in the city compared with college X students living in the country can be calculated. The null hypothesis for this comparison would be—

H_0: proportion of asthma$_{\text{students living in the city}}$

= proportion of asthma$_{\text{students living in the country}}$

or H_0: RR = 1

TABLE 6-3. **Interpretation of Relative Risk**

Relative Risk	Association between Exposure and Outcome
1	No association
< 1	Negative association/Decreased risk
> 1	Positive association/Increased risk

Using the data presented in Table 6-2, the relative risk can be calculated. The cumulative incidence has already been calculated in example 6-3. The relative risk is merely a ratio of $CI_{exposed}$ over $CI_{unexposed}$.

$$RR = \frac{CI_{exposed}}{CI_{unexposed}} = \frac{A/A + B}{C/C + D}$$

$$RR = \frac{200/1400}{100/1300} = 1.86$$

Students in college X who live in the city have 1.86 times the risk of developing asthma than students in college X who live in the country.

The 95% confidence intervals of the relative risk can be calculated. The confidence intervals determine the reliability of the risk estimate obtained in the sample. As mentioned in Chapter 5, confidence intervals are defined as the range within which the true effect lies with a certain degree of assurance. The confidence interval for a relative risk is calculated as follows:

$$CI = RRe^{\{\pm z\sqrt{\text{variance}(\ln RR)}\}}$$

The confidence interval can be calculated at various degrees of confidence. Confidence intervals are most frequently reported at the 95% level, corresponding with a z-value of 1.96. Therefore, the 95% confidence interval will be calculated as follows:

$$95\% \; CI = RRe^{\{\pm 1.96\sqrt{\text{variance}(\ln RR)}\}}$$

The confidence intervals, like the p-value, provide information regarding the statistical significance of the result. When interpreting the confidence intervals around a relative risk, a 95% confidence interval that includes 1 (the null hypothesis), is not statistically significant ($p > 0.05$). As noted in Chapter 5, the confidence intervals provide other valuable information pertaining to the reliability of the risk estimate. The wider the confidence intervals, the less reliable the risk estimate. However, the width of the confidence intervals is a function of the sample size; therefore, the smaller the sample size, the larger the confidence intervals. As discussed previously, a 95% confidence interval means that, if a study were conducted 100 times, the true measure of association (e.g., relative risk) would fall within the intervals 9.5 times. In other words, the investigator may have 95% assurance, or confidence, that the true measure of association (e.g., relative risk) lies within the confidence interval.

Consider the results of three different studies. The relative risk and the corresponding 95% confidence interval for each study were as follows:

$$\text{Study 1: RR} = 2.2; 95\% \text{ CI } (1.8, 2.6)$$

$$\text{Study 2: RR} = 2.2; 95\% \text{ CI } (1.1, 3.3)$$

$$\text{Study 3: RR} = 2.2; 95\% \text{ CI } (0.9, 3.0)$$

Note that all three studies derived the same relative risk, but the 95% confidence interval for the three studies were very different. Studies 1 and 2 show a statistically significant result because the number 1 is not included within the bounds of the 95% confidence interval; therefore the p-values associated with both study 1 and study 2 are ≤ 0.05. The 95% confidence interval for study 1 is narrower than the 95% confidence interval for study 2; therefore, there is more reliability in the relative risk estimate from study 1 than study 2. Study 3 does not show a statistically significant result because the number 1 is included within the bounds of the 95% confidence interval; therefore the p-value corresponding to study 3 is > 0.05. In other words, even though the relative risk is 2.2, the confidence interval indicate that the RR could be 1 (the null hypothesis) or even less than 1 (0.9).

Odds Ratio

The odds ratio (OR) is a means of estimating the relative risk in case-control studies. In case-control studies, subjects are chosen based on disease status and then compared for rates of exposure. Because the subjects are initially chosen based on whether they have the disease, the investigator cannot estimate the incidence of disease. Subjects either have the disease or do not have the disease at the onset of a case-control study. Because the relative risk is merely a ratio of two incidences, the relative risk is not useful in the context of a case-control study. Instead, the odds ratio is used to estimate the relative risk in a case-control study. The 2 × 2 contingency table can be used to derive the odds ratio. The odds ratio is calculated as follows:

$$OR = \frac{A/B}{C/D} \quad \text{or}$$

$$OR = \frac{AD}{BC}$$

The null hypothesis when using the odds ratio states, $H_0: OR = 1$.

The OR is interpreted in the same manner as the RR. As seen in Table 6-4, $OR = 1$ is the null hypothesis and means that there is no association between

TABLE 6-4. Interpretation of Odds Ratio

Odds Ratio	Association between Exposure and Outcome
1	No association
< 1	Negative association/Decreased risk
> 1	Positive association/Increased risk

exposure and outcome. OR < 1 suggests a protective effect or a decreased risk. OR > 1 suggests an increased risk of outcome associated with the exposure.

Example 6-6

In the context of a case-control design, the odds ratio for college X students can be determined using data from Table 6-2.

$$OR = \frac{AD}{BC}$$

$$OR = \frac{200\,(1200)}{1200\,(100)}$$

$$OR = 2$$

College X students who live in the city are 2 times as likely to have asthma than college X students who do not live in the city.

The 95% confidence interval for the odds ratio can be calculated as follows:

$$95\%\ CI\ OR = ORe^{\pm z\sqrt{1/a+1/b+1/c+1/d}} \quad \text{or}$$

$$95\%\ CI = \left(\frac{AD}{BC}\right)e^{\pm z\sqrt{1/a+1/b+1/c+1/d}}$$

The 95% confidence interval for the odds ratio is interpreted in exactly the same way as the 95% confidence interval for the relative risk. Remembering that the odds ratio obtained in the sample is merely an estimate and not the absolute risk in the population at large, the 95% confidence interval indicates that the investigator can be 95% confident that the true odds ratio lies within the bounds of the confidence interval.

Example 6-7

The 95% confidence interval for the odds ratio determined in example 6-5 is calculated as follows:

$$95\%\ CI_{OR} = \left(\frac{200 \times 1200}{1200 \times 100}\right)e^{\pm 1.96\sqrt{1/200+1/1200+1/100+1/1200}}$$

$$95\%\ CI = (1.55, 2.58)$$

The investigator can be 95% confident that the true odds ratio lies between 1.55 and 2.58. Or, if the study were conducted 100 times, 95 times out of 100 the OR would fall between 1.55 and 2.58 95 times.

It can be concluded that there is an association between living in the city and developing asthma. It cannot be concluded that living in the city causes asthma. Remember, observational studies never show causation; observational studies show only associations between exposures and outcomes.

Interpretation of Risk Estimates

In addition to the 95% confidence interval corresponding to a particular risk estimate, other factors should be considered when assessing the utility of a risk estimate. First, it is important to consider the baseline risk of developing the outcome of interest. For example, assume that taking drug A increases the risk of developing disease B by 2 (RR = 2). If the incidence of disease B is 0.0001%, then increasing the risk of developing disease B by 2 leads to an incidence of 0.002%, still an arguably low risk. However, if the incidence of disease B is 10%, then increasing the risk of developing disease B by 2 leads to an incidence of 20%. Therefore, large risk estimates may have no significant public health effect if the incidence of the outcome of interest is very low.

Second, it is also important to consider all of the variables that could potentially be related to the outcome of interest. In the college X example, we considered only one exposure in relation to one outcome. There are, in fact, many other factors that could contribute to the development of asthma—allergies and smoking, for example. As discussed previously, these factors are called *confounders,* and they exist in every study. They are variables that are related to the exposure and may contribute to the development of disease.

Confounding can be handled by one of two methods: excluding subjects with known confounding attributes from the study or controlling for the confounding variables in statistical analyses (e.g., stratification, multivariate analysis). Certain confounders are best handled by exclusion, and other confounders are best handled by statistical analysis. Excluding all subjects with a potential confounder limits both the number of subjects eligible for the study and the generalizablity of the study results.

In the college X example, students living in the city had higher rates of asthma. There are numerous reasons that living in the city may increase risk of developing asthma. For example, pollution, which is much higher in the city than in the country, may be confounding the effect of city living in the development of asthma. One way to test for pollution as a confounder is to divide the city residents into areas of high and low pollution and to compare the rates of asthma in the two areas. If the high-pollution area of the city has a higher rate of asthma than the low-pollution area of the city, then pollution would be a confounder in this study.

When assessing the role of confounding in a study, it is important to first identify all of the potential confounders. If the investigator identified all of the potential confounders and adequately handled them with either exclusion or statistical analysis, then one may feel confident in the risk estimate obtained from the study. However, if there are potential confounders that were not identified by the investigator, then one may be legitimately concerned that a confounder, rather than the exposure measured in the study, is responsible for the results obtained in the study.

Attributable Risk or Risk Difference

Attributable risk (AR) or risk difference (RD) is another measure of risk used in studies. The attributable risk provides information on the absolute effect of the exposure. Attributable risk describes the excess risk of disease in those exposed compared with those who were unexposed. Attributable risk is calculated as follows:

$$AR = CI_{exposed} - CI_{unexposed} \quad \text{or}$$

$$AR = \frac{A}{A + B} - \frac{C}{C + D}$$

Attributable risk allows the investigator to determine how morbidity and mortality are affected by removing the exposure. An attributable risk of 0 is equal to the null hypothesis and means there is no association between exposure and outcome. The attributable risk becomes important for agencies attempting to appropriate monies to reduce exposures. The attributable risk provides information on the type of effect that can be achieved by decreasing or eliminating the exposure.

The null hypothesis for using the attributable risk states, H_0: AR = 0. This is slightly different from the null hypothesis tested in regard to the relative risk and the odds ratio. Remember, the null hypothesis states that the two groups are equal. The relative risk and the odds ratio are proportions and are derived by dividing the risk in one group by the risk in another group. Therefore, if the two groups have equal risk, then the relative risk or the odds ratio is equal to 1 and the null hypothesis is accepted. In contrast, the attributable risk is a difference, not a proportion. The attributable risk is derived by subtracting the risk in one group from the risk in the other group. Therefore, if the two groups have equal risk, then the attributable risk is equal to 0, and the null hypothesis is accepted.

Example 6-8

The attributable risk for college X students can be calculated using data from Table 6-2 as follows:

$$AR = CI_{exposed} - CI_{unexposed}$$

$$AR = \frac{A}{A + B} - \frac{C}{C + D}$$

$$AR = \frac{200}{1400} - \frac{100}{1300}$$

$$AR = 0.06593$$

The attributable risk can be expressed in words by stating that the excess occurrence of asthma in the city attributable to living in the city is 6593 cases per 100,000. In other words, if living in the city causes asthma, then 6593 cases of asthma per 100,000 subjects could be eliminated if living in the city were eliminated.

The 95% confidence interval can be calculated for the attributable risk. As stated previously, the 95% confidence interval provides information on both the statistical significance and the reliability of the risk estimate. When interpreting the 95% confidence interval around the attributable risk, the number 0 cannot be included in the confidence interval if the result is to be considered statistically significant.

Consider the results of three studies. The attributable risk and the corresponding 95% confidence interval for each study are as follows:

$$\text{Study 1: AR} = 0.3; 95\% \text{ CI } (0.2, 0.4)$$
$$\text{Study 2: AR} = 0.3; 95\% \text{ CI } (0.1, 0.5)$$
$$\text{Study 3: AR} = 0.3; 95\% \text{ CI } (-0.8, 0.7)$$

Note that all three of the studies derived the same attributable risk, but the 95% confidence interval for the three studies are very different. Studies 1 and 2 show a statistically significant result because the number 0 is not included within the bounds of the 95% confidence interval; therefore the p-values associated with both study 1 and study 2 are ≤ 0.05. The 95% confidence interval for study 1 are narrower than the 95% confidence interval for study 2; therefore, there is more reliability in the attributable risk estimate from study 1 than study 2. Study 3 does not show a statistically significant result because the number 0 is included within the bounds of the 95% confidence interval; therefore, the p-value corresponding to study 3 is > 0.05.

Attributable Risk Percent

The attributable risk can then be converted to the attributable risk percent (AR%), which may be easier to interpret. The attributable risk percent provides an estimate of the proportion of the disease among the exposed that is attributable to the exposure. Like the attributable risk, it provides information pertaining to the proportion of the disease in the exposed group that could be prevented by eliminating the exposure. The attributable risk percent is calculated as follows:

$$AR\% = \frac{CI_{exposed} - CI_{unexposed}}{CI_{exposed}} \times 100$$

$$AR\% = \frac{\dfrac{A}{A+B} - \dfrac{C}{C+D}}{\dfrac{A}{A+B}} \times 100$$

EXAMPLE 6-9

The attributable risk percent for college X students can be calculated using data from Table 6-2 ás follows:

$$AR\% = \frac{CI_{exposed} - CI_{unexposed}}{CI_{exposed}} \times 100$$

$$AR\% = \frac{\dfrac{A}{A + B} - \dfrac{C}{C + D}}{\dfrac{A}{A + B}} \times 100$$

$$AR\% = \frac{\dfrac{200}{1400} - \dfrac{100}{1300}}{\dfrac{200}{1400}} \times 100$$

$$AR\% = 46\%$$

If living in the city causes asthma, then approximately 46% of asthma among subjects living in the city can be attributed to living in the city and could, therefore, be eliminated if the subjects did not live in the city.

Number Needed to Treat

The *number needed to treat* (NNT) is an estimate used primarily in pharmacoeconomical studies. This estimate represents the number of patients one would need to treat to prevent one clinical event. Like the attributable risk, the number needed to treat is used by administrators to allocate health resources. It can be calculated as follows:

$$\mathbf{NNT} = \frac{1}{AR}$$

EXAMPLE 6-10

Using the data in example 6-8, we can calculate the number needed to treat as follows:

$$NNT = \frac{1}{AR}$$

$$AR = 0.06593$$

$$NNT = \frac{1}{0.06593} = 15.17$$

To prevent 1 person from developing asthma, 15.17 people would have to move from the city.

Summary

In conclusion, measures of risk allow the quantification of degree of risk associated with any number of exposures. Risk estimates are point estimates, the estimates obtained in the particular study population. Therefore, risk estimates may or may not represent the true, or actual, risk that exists in the general population. When evaluating risk estimates, it is important to consider the baseline risk of developing the disease. In addition, it is important to evaluate the confidence intervals around the risk estimate to determine the stability of the risk estimate. Confidence intervals that include the null hypothesis will never be statistically significant. Finally, it is important to consider other factors that may be responsible for the disease, including confounding variables. If confounders are not eliminated by study design through exclusion criteria, then they should be considered in the statistical analyses.

References

1. Pahor M, Guralnik JM, Corti M-C, et al. Calcium-channel blockade and incidence of cancer in aged populations. *Lancet.* 1996;348:493–497.

2. Pahor M, Guralnik JM, Salive ME, Corti M-C, Carbonin P, Havlik RJ. Do calcium channel blockers increase the risk of cancer? *Am J Hypertens.* 1996; 9:695–699.

3. Fitzpatrick AL, Daling JR, Furberg CD, Krommal RA, Weissfeld JL. Use of calcium channel blockers and breast carcinoma risk in postmenopausal women. *Cancer.* 1997;80:1438–1447.

4. Jick H, Jick S, Derby LE, Vasilakis C, Myrs MW, Meier CR. Calcium channel blockers and risk of cancer. *Lancet.* 1997;349:525–528.

5. Rosenberg L, Rao S, Palmer JR, et al. Calcium channel blockers and the risk of cancer. *JAMA.* 1998;279(13):1000–1004.

Study Questions

1. Define each of the following risk measures as either a prevalence, a cumulative incidence, or an incidence rate:

   a. Each year, 2.2 million new cases of cancer are diagnosed, including about 1 million new cases of skin cancer.

   b. Investigators reported in a recent cross-sectional study of 425 HIV-positive subjects receiving antiretroviral therapy that 11 subjects showed signs or symptoms of hepatotoxicity.

   c. In 1997, an estimated 64,207 people sustained nonfatal firearm-related injuries and were treated in U.S. hospital emergency rooms.

   d. In 1997, 33% of firearm-related injuries resulted in death.

e. A recent cohort study comparing ACE-inhibitor users to ACE-inhibitor nonusers showed that 50 ACE-inhibitor users developed a cough during 2470 person-years of follow-up.

2. Consider the following hypothetical study: On January 20, 2000, an investigator enrolled 1700 subjects in a study. Subjects who had had a myocardial infarction (MI) in the past year were compared to subjects who have not had an MI within the past year for history of coronary artery disease (CAD).

a. What type of study design is the investigator using?

b. Assume the following results: 1700 subjects were enrolled in the study. Of these subjects 100 who had had an MI also had a history of CAD. Twenty subjects had had an MI but did not have a history of CAD. A total of 700 subjects in the study had no history of CAD. Calculate the risk of having an MI for subjects with a history of CAD compared with subjects without a history of CAD. In other words, calculate either the odds ratio or relative risk, whichever is more appropriate. Express the odds ratio in your own words.

c. Calculate the 95% confidence intervals for the risk estimate calculated above. Express the 95% confidence intervals in your own words.

d. Is the risk estimate calculated above statistically significant? Explain.

e. Comment on the reliability of the risk estimate calculated above.

f. List three potential confounders to be considered in this study.

3. Convert the following statements into relative risk figures:

a. Men who are losing the hair on the crowns of their heads have a 36% greater risk of experiencing heart problems, including heart attacks and bypass surgery.

b. Pravastatin use can reduce the risk of first heart attacks by 31%.

Chapter 7

Screening and Diagnostic Testing

Screening and diagnostic testing are not primary activities of pharmacoepidemiology, but they are important functions of both public health and epidemiology. Assessing the usefulness of a screening or diagnostic test is based on the sensitivity, the specificity, and the predictive value of the test's results compared with what is actually occurring. One example of testing that is very pertinent to drug use are tests (e.g., urine, hair, breath) designed to assess whether a person has been using certain psychoactive drugs. But, first, there must be a discussion of data quality, including the concepts of validity and reliability with regard to research results.

Data Quality: Validity and Reliability

One of the most important aspects of research results pertains to their validity. Interpretation of research results begins with judgments about their accuracy. The *validity* of a measure refers to the degree to which it actually measures what it is designed to measure. *Internal validity* is the extent to which the results of a study accurately reflect the situation in reality, whereas *external validity* is the extent to which the study's results are applicable to other populations.

One way of appraising validity is to compare a set of criteria known or believed to be close to reality. In the absence of this kind of criteria, it would be helpful to know the results of any follow-up study showing association between the results of the test and subsequent events (e.g., diseases, drug use problems). Associations between known criteria and other variables are one way of appraising validity, but there are others: developing a consensus of experts' opinions; using a set of questions that covers all of the essential components of what they purport to measure (i.e., content validity); and using measures that give the same results when repeated (i.e., reliability of the measure).

Reliability is defined as the degree of stability exhibited when a measurement is repeated under identical conditions. In other words, reliability refers to the degree to which a measure or result can be replicated. Lack of reliability may arise from divergence among observers or instruments of measurement or from the instability of the attribute being measured. Reliability is not a guarantee of validity. It is usually measured by performing two or more independent measurements and comparing the findings. The goals of such independent measurements can include determination of whether the observers vary on their measurements (interrater variation), there are differences between measurements made by the same observer at different times (intrarater variation), the measurement instruments differ, or the attribute being measured is itself unstable.

Bias is systematic error in a study that leads to distortion of the results. When bias occurs, the study's results do not accurately reflect reality. Bias can result during the selection of a study sample or during information and data collection, or it can result from the influence of a confounding variable. Selection bias is an especially important problem in case-control studies. In cohort studies and clinical trials, a major form of selection bias is the proportion of subjects or patients who are lost to follow-up. Information bias, or misclassification, as discussed in Chapter 2, can occur when there is random or systematic inaccuracy in measurement. Two types of information bias are *recall bias* (the ability of study subjects to remember previous events or exposures) and *interviewer bias* (collectors of data, such as interviewers, influence the results by their means of data collection).

As previously discussed, a *confounding variable* influences the relationship between an independent variable (e.g., exposure, risk factor) and a dependent variable (e.g., disease, study outcome), altering the true relationship between them. A potential confounding variable must be associated with the disease or outcome of interest in the absence of the exposure, and it must be associated with the exposure but not as a consequence of the exposure. Potential confounding variables are usually limited to established risk factors of the disease under study. The impact of confounding variables can be managed through (1) the design of the study, by matching subjects on the confounding variable or by restricting the sample to limited levels of the confounding variable; or (2) the analysis of study data, by evaluating the extent of confounding through stratification of data or by using multivariate analyses.

For example, it is known from many studies that the risk of myocardial infarction (MI) is associated with obesity and that cholesterol levels also are associated with obesity. A new case-control study is performed, and the results show that 80% of patients who had an MI also had high cholesterol levels, whereas only 20% of control subjects had high cholesterol levels. Thus, the results of this study appear to show that high cholesterol levels are associated with a 4 times increased risk of MI (RR = 80%/20% = 4). If this association, however, were examined separately for obese and nonobese subjects, then there would be a different result. For instance, among obese subjects in this study, 90% of the cases and 85% of the controls had high cholesterol levels (RR = 90%/85% = 1.1). Among the nonobese subjects, 20% of the cases and 15% of the controls had high cholesterol levels (RR = 20%/15% = 1.3). A high cholesterol level and its relationship to the risk of MI are essentially the same for obese and nonobese subjects. In this example, obesity was the confounding variable that altered the apparent relationship between cholesterol levels and the risk of having an MI.

Purpose of Screening and Diagnostic Testing

The purpose of screening populations is to detect as many people with a disease (cases) as possible. Screening and disease detection are very important aspects of public health. Screening programs are one tool used to prevent disease in a population. A *screening test* can be defined as the use of quick and simple testing procedures to identify and separate people who are apparently well but who may be at risk for a disease from those who probably do not have the disease. Screening is used to identify people suspected of having a disease and, if there is a positive result, the person can be given more definitive diagnostic studies and examination. Factors that are important to consider when planning a screening program for large populations are listed in Table 7-1.

Screening is sometimes confused with diagnosis, but it should be seen as a precursor to diagnosis. Most screening tests, such as vision tests, blood pressure, pap smear, blood tests, and glaucoma checks, are given to large groups or whole populations. Screening tests have cutoff points that are used to determine which people have the disease and which people are free of the disease. *Diagnosis* is applied to a patient on a one-to-one basis by a physician. Diagnosis may use the results of screening tests as well as signs, symptoms, and other subjective measures. A diagnosis can confirm or refute a screening test result, and it also can help to establish the validity, sensitivity, and specificity of the test.

For instance, the estimated probability of a positive diagnosis of breast cancer (in a 55-year-old woman) can be related to different screening and diagnostic test-

TABLE 7-1. **Considerations in Planning a Screening Program**

The disease or condition being screened should be a major medical problem.

Acceptable treatment should be available for individuals with the disease who are discovered through the screening process.

Access to health care facilities and services for follow-up should be available.

The disease should have a recognized course, with early and late stages of the disease being identifiable.

Tests and testing procedures should be acceptable to the general population.

The natural history of the disease should be adequately understood.

Policies and procedures should be determined to know who should be referred for further testing or treatment.

The process should be simple enough to encourage large groups of people to participate.

Screening should not be an occasional activity; it should be conducted on an ongoing basis.

---

ing results. Based on a normal breast examination (a type of screening), the estimated probability that this woman will actually develop breast cancer is almost 0 (less than 0.5%). If the woman's sister or mother were previously diagnosed with breast cancer, then the estimated probability would increase to 1%. A positive mammogram (another screening test) would increase the likelihood of that woman developing cancer to about 15%, whereas a palpable breast lump would lead to an estimated probability of cancer of between 20% and 40%. A positive fine-needle aspiration test would increase the likelihood of developing cancer to around 65%. The basic idea of using these various tests is to increase (toward 100%) or decrease (toward 0%) the estimated probability of disease development for a person so that the clinician can make a correct diagnosis of disease as early as possible.

Sensitivity, Specificity, and Predictive Value

It would be ideal if medical tests were always correct. In reality, however, every test is fallible. Consider a test that has only positive or negative results. The four possibilities, then, in the test results are true positive, false positive, true negative, and false negative. The true occurrence of disease is determined by the most definitive diagnostic method then available. It may be a cellular examination, a biopsy, a biochemical marker, or the identification of specific signs and symptoms.

Two basic aspects of screening tests are their accuracy, or validity, and their reproducibility, or precision. People who test positive for a disease and who actually have the disease are called *true positives*. Those who test positive but do not have the disease are called *false positives*. Those who test negative and do not have the disease are called *true negatives,* and people who test negative but have the disease are called *false negatives*. Sensitivity and specificity are determined from these results. Screening tests are used to classify individuals as having or not having a specific disease. The *sensitivity* of a test is the proportion of correct results among people who actually have the disease, whereas the *specificity* of a test is the proportion of correct results among people who are actually free of the disease.

Two other measures are helpful in determining the value of a screening test— the predictive value of positive test results and the predictive value of negative test results. *Positive predictive value* is the proportion of people actually with the disease among all of the people with positive test results. It measures the probability that a person with a positive result has the disease. It also provides an indication of how much cost and effort will be required to offer a screening program. *Negative predictive value* is the proportion of people free of the disease among all of the people with negative test results, or the probability that a person with a negative test result is free of the disease. It also is another measure of validity.

Sensitivity (Sen): probability that a person who actually has the condition will have a positive (abnormal) test result.

$$\text{Sen} = \frac{\text{number of people with disease who test positive}}{\substack{\text{number of people with disease who test positive } + \\ \text{number of people with disease who test negative}}}$$

Specificity (SPE): probability that a person who actually does not have the condition will have a negative (normal) test result.

$$SPE = \frac{\text{number of people without disease who test negative}}{\text{number of people without disease who test negative} + \text{number of people without disease who test positive}}$$

Positive Predictive Value (PV+): probability that a person with a positive (abnormal) test result actually has the disease under study.

$$PV+ = \frac{\text{number of people with disease who test positive}}{\text{number of people with disease who test positive} + \text{number of people without disease who test positive}}$$

Negative Predictive Value (PV−): probability that a person with a negative (normal) test result actually does not have the disease.

$$PV- = \frac{\text{number of people without disease who test negative}}{\text{number of people without disease who test negative} + \text{number of people with disease who test negative}}$$

Sensitivity and specificity are not absolute values, as each use of a test might produce a slightly different response. Sensitivity and specificity for each test are determined through use over a span of time. Long-term use of a test establishes reliability and reveals the test's shortcomings. There is a relationship between sensitivity and specificity in terms of setting the cutoff point (i.e., defining the "normal" test value or limit for a positive test result). (See Figure 7-1.)

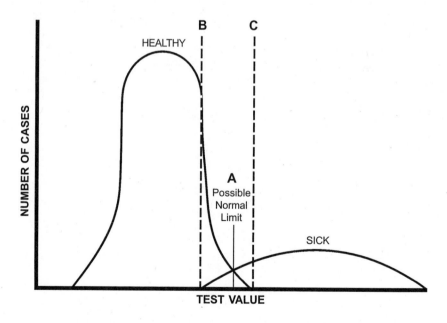

Figure 7-1. Relationship between sensitivity and specificity.

In this case, the test can have a range of values, and it becomes important to decide where the cutoff for positive versus negative test results will be set. One possible normal limit might be set at point A. With this choice of value, the test will correctly identify most of the sick people in a population (true positives), but it will miss a small proportion of the sick subjects in a population (false negatives). In contrast, the test will not identify most of the healthy people as having the disease (true negatives), but it will indicate that a few healthy people have the disease (false positives). Moving the cutoff limit of the test's value down to a lower number in its range (point B) will change the results. In this situation, the test will correctly identify all of the sick people in a population but at a cost. More healthy people will be identified as having the disease, when, in reality, they do not. In this study, moving the cutoff number down increased the test's sensitivity but decreased its specificity. The cutoff limit of the test's value could also be moved up to a higher number in its range (point C). Although none of the healthy people then would be identified as having the disease, many more sick people would be missed by the test, showing negative results (a normal test value). Moving the cutoff number up increased the test's specificity but decreased its sensitivity. Determining the best cutoff level or limit for a screening test is one of the most important considerations in planning and performing a screening program.

The predictive value of a screening test is determined by both its validity and characteristics of the population being tested, especially the prevalence of preclinical disease. The higher the prevalence of a disease in a population, the more the sensitivity and the specificity of a test affect its predictive value. The higher the prevalence of a disease in a population, the more likely it is that higher numbers of true positives should occur. With more sensitivity and higher predictive value, the number of false positives should be lower.

A case example showing the use of the enzyme-linked immunosorbent assay (ELISA) test to screen for the antibody to HIV portrays these relationships.[1] In a large blood donation program, 1,000,000 people were tested in the general population, which has an HIV prevalence of 0.04% (see Table 7-2). The ELISA test has a test sensitivity of 95% and a test specificity of 98%.

TABLE 7-2. **Predictive Value of ELISA Test in General Population**

ELISA Test	HIV Diagnosed	Healthy (No HIV)	Totals
Positive	380 (A)	19,992 (B)	20,372
Negative	20 (C)	979,608 (D)	979,628
Totals	400	999,600	1,000,000

TABLE 7-3. **Predictive Value of ELISA Test in Addict Population**

ELISA Test	HIV Diagnosed	Healthy (No HIV)	Totals
Positive	95 (A)	18 (B)	113
Negative	5 (C)	882 (D)	887
Totals	100	900	1000

The calculations for positive and negative predictive value are as follows:

$$PV+ = \frac{A}{A+B} = \frac{380}{380+19{,}992} = \frac{380}{20{,}372} = 1.9\%$$

$$PV- = \frac{D}{C+D} = \frac{979{,}608}{20+979{,}608} = \frac{979{,}608}{979{,}628} = 99.9\%$$

In this population, the positive predictive value of the test is determined to be 1.9% (many false negatives), whereas the negative predictive value is 99.9% (very few false positives).

In the donation program, 1000 intravenous (IV) drug users, with a much higher HIV prevalence of 10%, were tested (see Table 7-3). The ELISA test was the same, with the same sensitivity and specificity as in the previous example of the general population.

The calculations for positive and negative predictive value are as follows:

$$PV+ = \frac{A}{A+B} = \frac{95}{113} = 84.1\%$$

$$PV- = \frac{D}{C+D} = \frac{882}{887} = 99.4\%$$

In this population, however, the positive predictive value increased considerably from 1.9% in the general population to 84.1% in the IV drug–using population. Many more IV drug users with HIV were correctly identified with a positive test; thus, there were many fewer false negatives. The negative predictive value of the test was reduced very little, from 99.9% to 99.4%, which means a few more IV drug users were identified as not having HIV when, in fact, they do have HIV (more false negatives). This situation is very problematic, as some drug users might believe they do not have HIV when they are sick.

Summary

Screening tests are important tools in public health efforts to prevent or identify and treat disease in a population.[2] Once the basic technique or procedure for a screening test has been developed, its sensitivity, specificity, and predictive value must be determined. This information will assist public health professionals in deciding appropriate values for indicating positive versus negative test results and in the planning and implementation of the screening program.

References

1. Duh M. Screening as a diagnostic tool. Unpublished handout and case study presented at: Massachusetts College of Pharmacy & Health Sciences; March 1997; Boston.

2. Hennekens CH, Buring JE. *Epidemiology in Medicine*. Boston: Little, Brown & Co.; 1987.

Study Questions

1. Definitions:

    a. validity

    b. reliability

    c. bias

    d. confounding variable

    e. screening test

    f. sensitivity

    g. specificity

    h. positive predictive value

    i. negative predictive value

2. Describe the relationship between sensitivity and specificity in terms of setting the cutoff point (i.e., defining the "normal" test value or limit for defining a positive result).

3. Describe the relationship between test validity and the prevalence of a disease with regard to the test's predictive value.

4. A new hair test has been developed to identify cocaine users. To determine whether the test is valid, a study is performed on 10,000 people. The results of both the hair test and a blood test for the presence of cocaine in these 10,000 people are presented in Table 7-4. Determine the value of the new hair test by calculating its sensitivity and specificity, and discuss the real-life implications of these results if the hair test were used.

TABLE 7-4. Value of Hair Test for Cocaine Use

Hair Test	Cocaine-Positive Blood Test	Cocaine-Negative Blood Test	Totals
Positive	475 (A)	475 (B)	950
Negative	25 (C)	9025 (D)	9050
Totals	500	9500	10,000

Chapter 8

Post-Marketing Surveillance

Post-marketing surveillance (PMS) is the identification and collection of information regarding medications after their approval by the U.S. Food and Drug Administration (FDA). Systematic PMS of drugs began in the early 1970s and has increased substantially since then. The monitoring of drugs after their approval has become necessary for many reasons. In the 1950s and 1960s, there were fewer drugs available and, thus, fewer drugs to monitor. Today, drugs are being developed and consumed at increasingly high rates. Other factors contributing to the need for PMS include changes in the FDA's approval process. As discussed in Chapter 4, this lengthy process has been criticized. The FDA has responded by developing channels and opportunities for patients in need to obtain critical drugs. As a result, the dangers associated with use of some drugs may not be determined in the premarketing phase.

PMS is conducted by various types of organizations and agencies, including pharmaceutical manufacturers, universities, government agencies, private companies, and consumer advocacy groups. The purpose of conducting PMS may differ, depending on the perspective of the individuals conducting the surveillance. This chapter provides an overview of PMS, including its definition and purpose, available methods, and several examples of the application of PMS in clinical practice.

Definition and Purposes

Since the drug approval process involves phase I, II, and III trials, post-marketing trials are sometimes referred to as *phase IV trials*. PMS involves systematic monitoring of medications as they are used in real-life scenarios, as opposed to the controlled settings of pre-marketing trials, where study conditions are tightly controlled. Although randomized, RT clinical trials, which minimize variability, are useful in assessing the efficacy of one drug versus another, they do not provide adequate information on a drug's effects after it is released for general use.

PMS provides valuable information on the use of drugs in special patient populations, which is information not easily obtainable from pre-marketing studies. Randomized clinical trials conducted before marketing include only subjects who meet defined inclusion and exclusion criteria, thus creating a homogenous study population. The population of potential users after the drug is released is very different from the population studied in the pre-marketing phase. For example, randomized clinical trials typically exclude from study participation women who are pregnant or breastfeeding; therefore, PMS is the only means of obtaining information on mutagenic and teratogenic effects of drugs in humans. Other special populations that benefit from PMS include the elderly and patients with multiple comorbidities. Like pregnant women, patients who are very old or very sick are excluded from premarketing trials. A drug may exhibit different effects when administered to a healthy 30-year-old patient versus an 85-year-old patient who has multiple health problems and is taking multiple medications.

PMS also allows for long-term monitoring of the effects of drugs. Due to cost and feasibility issues, randomized clinical trials conducted before marketing are short in duration. Thus, experience with drugs at the time of marketing is based on short observation periods. The drug may or may not continue to work as it did in the context of a clinical trial. Long-term use may result in adverse drug reactions or, alternatively, tolerance to the drug's effects.

PMS can detect rare adverse events that may not be detectable during clinical trials with inadequate sample sizes. Pre-marketing trials cannot detect adverse drug reactions that occur at rates of 1 in 10,000 or less.[1,2] For example, a study with 80% statistical power would require sample sizes of 161, 1610, and 16,095 subjects to detect adverse drug reactions occuring at frequencies of 1/100, 1/1000, and 1/10,000, respectively. Studies with less power would require smaller sample sizes to detect the same adverse drug reactions, whereas studies with greater power would require larger sample sizes to detect the same reactions. Rare adverse drug reactions can be identified, quantified, and studied using PMS methods.

PMS allows for the best description of drug use in the population at large. During premarketing trials, a drug is studied for effectiveness for one particular indication. When the drug is released onto the market, it may be used for numerous indications that were not studied in the pre-marketing phase. Other fixed parameters in randomized clinical trials include the dose and duration of therapy. After the drug is released onto the market, these parameters will vary drastically from those used in the pre-marketing studies. Therefore, knowledge gained from PMS allows for the broader application of medicines to special populations, for different indications, and at doses and durations not studied before marketing.

Types of Post-Marketing Surveillance

Many methods are used to monitor drugs after FDA approval. These methods include spontaneous reporting systems, case reports, case-control studies, cohort studies, randomized clinical trials, database research and monitoring, and meta-analyses. The decision-making process involved in choosing one method over another is similar to the process discussed in Chapters 3 and 4.

Spontaneous Reporting Systems

Spontaneous reporting systems are formal reporting systems designed to record, collate, and analyze the occurrence of adverse drug reactions. These systems are most commonly used to identify new reactions. If a practitioner (e.g., pharmacist, physician, nurse) suspects that a particular medication is associated with an adverse event observed during the course of caring for a patient, then he or she reports the adverse drug reaction to a formal reporting system. When several practitioners report adverse drug reactions to a central location, the data can then be reviewed and analyzed for trends. One practitioner observing one adverse drug reaction associated with a particular drug may not consider the adverse drug reaction to be significant or common, but several practitioners reporting the same adverse drug reaction to a central locale allows for the determination of its extent and seriousness.

Spontaneous reporting systems can be found at local, regional, and national levels. The Joint Commission for the Accreditation of Health Care Organizations requires that all health care institutions establish a formal adverse drug reaction reporting system. It is the responsibility of all practitioners to report suspected adverse drug reactions; however, the responsibility for the creation and maintenance of the reporting systems in health care institutions typically falls under the purview of the pharmacy department.

National reporting systems have been created to identify and monitor adverse drug reactions. In June 1993, the FDA launched the MEDWatch program to encourage adverse drug reaction reporting by practitioners and to identify the most serious adverse drug reactions with the greatest public health implications. The MEDWatch program is designed to serve as a central reporting agency for adverse drug reactions in the United States. Practitioners are encouraged to report to the FDA MEDWatch program any suspicions of serious adverse drug reactions. Suspected adverse drug reactions can be reported to the FDA by completing a form and forwarding it to the FDA via telephone, fax, the Internet, or U.S. mail.

The FDA is most interested in monitoring new medications and identifying previously unknown adverse drug reactions of a serious nature. The FDA defines *serious adverse drug reactions* as events resulting in death, life-threatening outcomes, disability, congenital anomaly, outcomes that require intervention to prevent permanent impairment, or outcomes requiring or prolonging hospitalization.[3]

The MEDWatch program, like all spontaneous reporting systems, solicits information on potentially confounding factors as well as the suspected drug and adverse drug reaction. Confounding information typically collected by spontaneous reporting systems includes age, gender, weight, race, allergies, past medical history, past surgical history, medication history, and social medication history. All confounding factors should be considered when determining the likelihood that the suspect drug actually caused the adverse drug reaction.

When the MEDWatch program receives a sufficient number of adverse drug reactions attributed to a particular drug, several enforcement options are available to the FDA. The agency can mandate the addition of information describing the newly detected adverse drug reaction to the drug's label or package insert. The FDA can also require the manufacturer to distribute letters to all registered physicians and pharmacists informing them about the newly identified adverse drug reaction. These letters typically include a description of the adverse drug reaction, its frequency of occurrence, risk factors, and instructions for monitoring the adverse drug reaction. Finally, the FDA can require the manufacturer to develop a formal surveillance program to monitor the rate and extent of adverse drug reaction occurrence; however, this step is uncommon and is typically suggested at the time of drug approval. If the drug's risks are determined to outweigh the benefits of the drug then the FDA can suggest withdrawal of the drug from the market.

Limitations of Spontaneous Reporting Systems. Spontaneous reporting systems are beneficial in providing the first warning of a potentially dangerous adverse drug reaction, but there are several limitations to these reporting systems. The spontaneous reporting system in the United States is voluntary. Unlike other countries, such as France, Norway, and Sweden, practitioners in the United States are not required to report adverse drug reactions to a national agency. Reporting rates in the United States, therefore, are much lower than in countries that mandate adverse drug reaction reporting. It is estimated that 10% of hospital admissions are related to adverse drug reactions and up to 20% of patients experience an adverse drug reaction while admitted to the hospital.

Adverse drug reaction reporting appears to be directly proportional to the duration of time a drug is on the market. Reporting is highest immediately after a new drug is released onto the market. In time, practitioners become familiar with the drug and cease to report adverse drug reactions associated with the drug.

The underreporting of adverse drug reactions makes it impossible to determine the number of patients who have actually experienced a particular reaction. It is also impossible to determine the number of patients who have used, or been exposed to, a particular medication. Without knowing the number of patients exposed to a drug or the number of patients who developed the adverse drug reaction, it is impossible to determine the incidence of the reaction. Therefore, the actual incidence of adverse drug reactions can never be determined through spontaneous reporting systems.

Other limitations of spontaneous reporting systems include lack of information about confounding factors. Although, the FDA MEDWatch program inquires about potential confounders (e.g., comorbidities, concurrent drug use), the reporter may not completely or accurately list all of them. Spontaneous reports are subject to observation and reporting bias. If a practitioner suspects that a particular drug causes a certain adverse drug reaction, then the practitioner may underreport other contributing factors associated with the reaction. In the context of multiple health problems and polypharmacy, it is difficult to determine the probability that the drug is actually responsible for the adverse event.

As mentioned in Chapter 6, any information obtained from a epidemiological study or surveillance program must be viewed in the context of the strengths and limitations of the study providing the information. Before the FDA takes serious action on a suspected adverse drug reaction, reliable information must be collected on the rate of occurrence of the reaction, its severity, and the likelihood that the drug actually caused it. The dissemination of spontaneous reports can sound unnecessary alarms if information in the report is lacking or incorrect.

Consider, for example, the spontaneous reports of fatal myocardial infarction (MI) associated with Viagra® use after the drug was approved by the FDA. Spontaneous reports were filed with the FDA and published as case reports in the medical literature. The reports were then communicated to the public via newspapers and television. Although the media reported the number of men who died from MI while taking Viagra®, no mention was made of the number of men who took Viagra® and did not experience an MI. In fact, millions of prescriptions were filled in the period immediately following FDA approval. Later, it was estimated that the incidence of fatal MI associated with Viagra was 49 per 1,000,000 prescriptions filled.[4] Upon closer examination of the cases, it was determined that the majority of men who suffered a Viagra®-associated MI had significant cardiac history and/or were taking medications that interacted with Viagra®.

Case Reports

Case reports and case series play a vital role in communicating previously unidentified uses and dangers of drugs because they allow practitioners to share their individual experiences in published medical literature. Case reports can serve the same role as spontaneous reports and warn practitioners of suspected adverse drug reactions. Case reports also offer the sharing of information about new indications or applications for drugs.

A striking example of the application of case reports and case series in PMS is the U.S. experience with the anorexant drug combination, phen-fen. The phen-fen combination is actually two separate drugs, phentermine and fenflufarmine, that are prescribed together to promote weight loss. Phentermine was approved by the FDA in 1971, and fenfluramine was approved in 1973. During the 20 years following approval, the drugs were prescribed individually, and patients received one drug or the other. Neither drug was widely used during this time period. Then, in the mid-1990s, it was determined that the combination use of the two drugs showed significant benefit in weight reduction. Phen-fen usage increased dramatically, thereafter. In 1996, more than 18,000,000 prescriptions were filled for the phen-fen combination.[5]

On August 28, 1997, Connolly and colleagues published a case series describing 24 young, overweight women with no prior history of cardiac disease who were diagnosed with valvular heart disease while taking the phen-fen combination.[6] Eight of the women in the case series also had pulmonary hypertension.[6] Many of the women required surgical intervention.[6] These cases alarmed practitioners, patients, and regulatory agencies. On September 5, 1997, fenfluramine was withdrawn from the market.

Case series can be very powerful tools. The phen-fen case series changed medical practice instantaneously. Practitioners began to screen patients using anorexant drugs for signs and symptoms of valvular heart disease and primary pulmonary hypertension. Practitioners also began eliciting information on cardiac risk factors before initiating anorexant drug therapy in new patients. In addition, practitioners reported many more anorexant-associated adverse drug reactions to the FDA, and more case reports were published in the medical literature.

This phen-fen case series also provided hypotheses and background information necessary to design and conduct more sophisticated observational studies to quantify the actual risk associated with anorexant use. Rich and colleagues reported a significant association between fenfluramine use for more than 6 months and the development of primary pulmonary hypertension.[7] They estimated an OR = 7.5 (95% CI = 1.7, 32.4).

Case-Control Studies

When PMS originated in the 1950s, it was via case reports and case series, but by the early 1970s, PMS had developed into more systematic methods. The first study design used to determine associations between drugs and adverse events was the case-control study. Initially, drug-related case-control studies were hospital based.[8]

As mentioned in Chapter 3, case-control studies are useful when the outcome of interest is rare, which is why case-control studies are often used to quantify rare adverse drug outcomes. Case-control studies are most commonly designed in a retrospective manner, as retrospective studies quickly provide answers at minimal expense.

In the early 1970s, the Boston Collaborative Drug Surveillance Program (BCDSP) was one of the first research organizations to conduct hospital-based case-control studies to assess drug safety. The BCDSP collaborated with the Group Health Cooperative of Puget Sound but eventually split into two separate groups now known as the Slone Epidemiology Unit and the BCDSP. Both groups continue to conduct valuable drug epidemiology research.

Cohort Studies

Prospective and retrospective cohort studies are employed in PMS. Cohort studies can be designed traditionally, such that a group of exposed subjects (e.g., medication users) and a group of unexposed subjects (e.g., medication nonusers) are compared to assess the occurrence of an outcome (e.g., adverse drug reaction).

Some of the largest and renown cohort studies include the Framingham Heart Study, the Physicians' Health Study, and the Nurses' Health Study. These cohorts were not designed solely to measure medication-related issues, but ultimately have provided a great deal of information in the area of drug epidemiology.

The Framingham Heart Study began in 1948 to determine risk factors associated with the development of cardiovascular disease.[9] The initial cohort consisted of 5209 male and female residents of Framingham, Massachusetts, ages 29 through 62.[9] The subjects were examined and interviewed on enrollment for various risk factors.[9] Every 2 years, the subjects would return for follow-up, which included physical examination, medical history, and laboratory tests.[9] Hundreds of studies have been conducted from this cohort, thereby providing a wealth of information on the prevention and treatment of cardiovascular disease. The cohort is ongoing and will provide further information on not only cardiovascular disease but also many other health problems.

The Physicians' and Nurses' Health studies are cohort studies similar to the Framingham Heart Study; however, subjects in these cohorts are chosen based on profession, rather than geographic location. The Nurses' Health Study began in 1976 and enrolled 121,700 female registered nurses 30 through 55 years old.[10] Information in this study is obtained via questionnaires on enrollment and every 2 years thereafter.[10]

The Physicians' Health Study originated as a randomized clinical trial of low-dose aspirin versus beta-carotene for prevention of cardiovascular disease and cancer.[11] It began in 1982 and enrolled 22,071 male physicians.[11] The subjects have since been followed in cohort studies evaluating many risk factors associated with various outcomes. Like the Nurses' Health Study, information is obtained via survey on enrollment and every 2 years thereafter. Both the Nurses' Health Study and the Physicians' Health Study have identified multiple dietary, social, and medication characteristics associated with disease occurrence and prevention. A similar cohort study following female physicians is ongoing.[12]

Other cohort designs used in PMS follow only the exposed individuals (e.g., medication users) over time to identify and quantify adverse events. In this design, there is no comparison to medication nonusers. The FDA may suggest such a surveillance program during the drug approval process if a serious adverse event is identified during the pre-marketing phase. The clozapine registry is an example of such a cohort. The incidence of agranulocytosis in pre-marketing trials was 1.3%. Given the serious nature of agranulocytosis, a registry was created to monitor patients receiving clozapine. Before initiating therapy, practitioners must obtain baseline white blood cell (WBC) levels on all patients. The patients and their corresponding baseline WBC levels are reported to the registry before the first dose of clozapine is dispensed. WBC levels must be measured and documented weekly for the drug to be dispensed to the patient, and all cases of agranulocytosis must be reported to the registry. The clozapine registry is a type of prospective cohort that allows for the safe use of a potentially dangerous drug.

Randomized Clinical Trials

Sample size, time, and cost considerations typically preclude randomized clinical trials from being used to identify or quantify adverse drug reactions. Recently, however, randomized clinical trials have been conducted for the purpose of establishing drug safety. As discussed in Chapter 4, the randomized clinical trial is considered the gold standard in epidemiological research. It is the only study design that can actually show that a particular drug caused a particular outcome, rather than merely suggesting an association between the exposure and the outcome. Mitchell and colleagues suggested that randomized clinical trials be used in situations when confounding by indication may occur, specifically in evaluating the safety of drugs used to treat nonserious conditions.[13] Mitchell and colleagues conducted a trial to assess the safety of pediatric ibuprofen versus acetaminophen in the treatment of febrile illness.[13] They evaluated 83,915 children and found no significant risks associated with short-term ibuprofen use in children.[13]

Database Research and Monitoring

Database research has gained popularity during the past several decades. Many health care organizations have automated all health care records such that outpatient visits, pharmacy records, and hospital admissions all are stored in one database. These databases can be used to evaluate associations between drug exposures and outcomes, providing all of the necessary information is recorded accurately in the database. Insurers and health maintenance organizations have realized the wealth of information stored in their databases and have conducted numerous PMS studies.

Although the databases provide a wealth of information, there are inherent limitations to database research. The accuracy of the data must be verified before conducting database research. Validation of some of the cases must be conducted. This validation is performed by taking a random sample (e.g., 10%) of cases generated by the computer and following up with either the patient or the practitioner to validate that the computer records are accurate and the patient truly has been diagnosed with the outcome of interest.

Other limitations to consider when conducting database research include lack of information on confounding factors. The database is a computerized version of the medical record. Information stored in the database was obtained through the routine medical care of patients; therefore, information on confounding factors may not be stored.

Meta-Analyses

Meta-analyses are studies that combine the results of two or more individual studies into one large study. They are also referred to as *systematic reviews*. Meta-analyses are useful when conflicting results are obtained in different studies or when studies had inadequate sample sizes.

Before conducting a meta-analysis, a literature search is conducted to identify all of the published studies on the topic of interest. Positive study results are more likely to be published than negative ones; therefore, an attempt must be made to locate unpublished studies. The studies are then reviewed for commonality. The studies included in the meta-analysis should be similar with regard to inclusion and exclusion criteria, doses used, and outcomes measured. Original data from all of the individual studies are combined into one large data set, and the pooled data are statistically analyzed.

A meta-analysis was conducted by Moore and colleagues in England to assess the effectiveness of topical nonsteroidal anti-inflammatory (NSAID) drugs.[14] Significant debate over the role of topical NSAIDs in the United Kingdom convinced the investigators to conduct a meta-analysis on the subject. The meta-analysis included 86 trials conducted to assess the efficacy of topical NSAIDs for the treatment of acute and chronic pain.[14] Meta-analysis of 10,160 subjects showed that topical NSAIDs were significantly more effective than placebo in the treatment of both acute and chronic pain.[14]

There are many limitations to meta-analyses. Whereas the design of the randomized clinical trial results in sample homogeneity, meta-analyses are inherently heterogeneous. The more variability among the individual studies used in the meta-analysis, the less reliable are the results. Studies included in meta-analyses must be carefully chosen. There should be similarity with regard to inclusion and exclusion criteria, definitions of outcomes, and the means by which the outcomes were measured. The methodologies of meta-analyses must be scrutinized before the results are applied to clinical practice.

Application of PMS: The Thalidomide Experience

One of the most significant drug-induced birth defects detected in PMS involved the use of thalidomide, a sedative widely used by pregnant women in Europe in the 1960s. At the time, thalidomide use was thought to be very safe, but the drug was later shown to be highly teratogenic, resulting in major birth defects. In the worst scenarios, infants were born with phocomelia, the absence or reduction of limbs. In some situations, flipper-like appendages grew in place of limbs. Case reports played a vital role in communicating the occurrence of thalidomide-associated phocomelia. The case reports led to case-control studies. It was estimated that 25% of babies exposed to thalidomide were born with some kind of birth defect.[15] Thalidomide was withdrawn from the European market, and the thalidomide experience propelled the United Kingdom to closely monitor drugs for safety both before and after marketing. Although thalidomide was never marketed in the United States, the European experience dramatically affected legislation regarding the drug approval process in the United States as well.

Years later, thanks to advances in PMS methods, thalidomide was introduced to the U.S. market. In 1998, thalidomide was approved by the FDA for the treatment of complications associated with leprosy. As part of the approval process, the FDA mandated strict surveillance of thalidomide use. A surveillance system was created that includes education of physicians, pharmacists, and patients regarding the risks associated with the drug. In addition, access to thalidomide is restricted to physicians and pharmacists who are registered in the program. Ongoing monitoring is required for patients to remain on thalidomide therapy. All adverse events are closely monitored and reported to the FDA. Despite the benefits thalidomide has shown, without PMS methods available today, thalidomide would never have been made available again to patients who can benefit from it.

Summary

Post-marketing surveillance plays an important role in identifying and measuring the effects and uses of drugs in clinical practice. All practitioners play a vital role in PMS. Practitioners should report serious adverse drug reactions to spontaneous reporting systems. The regulatory agencies cannot act on behalf of the public if they are not aware of the problem. Communication among practitioners via case reports and series will facilitate the dissemination of information regarding new uses and dangers of drugs. Observational and interventional studies can be used to monitor drugs after approval. All information gained from PMS must be reviewed in the context of the strengths and the limitations of the study design used and the quality of the data collected.

References

1. Anello C, O'Neill RT. Does research synthesis have a place in drug regulatory policy? Synopsis of issues: assessment of safety and postmarketing surveillance. *Clin Res Reg Aff*. 1996; 13:13–21.

2. Sills JIM, Tanner A, Milstein JB. Food and Drug Administration monitoring of adverse drug reactions. *Am J Hosp Pharmacy*. 1986;43:2764–2770.

3. Kessler DA. Introducing MEDWatch: A new approach to reporting medication and device adverse effects and product problems. *JAMA*. 1993; 269:2765–2768.

4. Mitka M. Some men who take Viagra die—Why? *JAMA*. 2000;283(5):590–592.

5. Langreth R. Critics claim diet clinics misuse obesity drugs. *Wall Street Journal*. March 31, 1997: B8.

6. Connolly HM, Crary JL, McGoon MD, et al. Valvular heart disease associated with fenfluramine-phentermine. *New Engl J Med*. 1997;337(9):581–588.

7. Rich S, Rubin L, Walker AM, Schneeweiss S, Abenhaim L. Anorexigens and pulmonary hypertension in the United States: Results from the surveillance of North American pulmonary hypertension. *Chest*. 2000;117(3):870–874.

8. Jick H, Vessey MP. Case-control studies in the evaluation of drug-induced illness. *Am J Epidemiol*. 1978;107:1–7.

9. Dawber TR, Meadors GF, Moore FE.Jr. Epidemiological approaches to heart disease: The Framingham Heart Study. *Am J Public Health*. 1951;41:279–286.

10. Willett WC, Stampfer MJ, Colditz GA, Rosner BA, Hennekens CH, Speizer FE. Dietary fat and the risk of breast cancer. *N Engl J Med*. 1987;316:22–28.

11. Steering Committee of the Physicians' Health Study Research Group. Final report on the aspirin component of the ongoing Physicians' Health Study. *N Engl J Med*. 1989;321:129–135.

12. Frank E. The women physicians' health study: Background information, objectives, and methods. *J Am Med Wom Assoc*. 1995;50:64–66.

13. Mitchell AA, Lesko SM. When a randomized controlled trial is needed to assess drug safety: The case of paediatric ibuprofen. *Drug Safety*. 1995;13(1):15–24.

14. Moore RA, Tramer MR, Carroll D, Wiffen PJ, McQuay HJ. Quantitative systematic review of topically applied non-steroidal anti-inflammatory drugs. *BMJ*. 2998;316:333–338.

15. Newman CGH. Teratogen update: Clinical aspects of thalidomide embryopathy—A continuing preoccupation. *Teratology*. 1985;32:133–134.

Study Questions

1. Define postmarketing surveillance.

2. List two limitations of premarketing trials in detecting adverse drug reactions.

3. List three methods used to monitor drugs after FDA approval.

4. List three limitations of spontaneous reporting systems in estimating adverse drug reactions.

5. List three actions the FDA can take after receipt of a serious adverse drug reaction associated with a particular drug.

Chapter 9

Principles of Pharmacoeconomics

William W. McCloskey, Pharm.D.

Pharmacoeconomics is the area of health care research that evaluates and compares the costs and outcomes associated with drug therapy.[1] Corresponding to recent awareness by the public of rising health care costs has been an increased interest in evaluating drugs' economic as well as clinical benefits. This interest is readily apparent by the steady growth in the number of pharmacoeconomical studies that have been published in the primary literature since the mid-1990s.[2]

Pharmacoeconomical research is primarily driven by the basic principle that financial resources are limited and that the organizational needs generally exceed available resources. Most pharmacy managers are constantly faced with doing "more with less," and choices must be made as to how best to allocate available dollars. Consequently, pharmacoeconomical studies help provide data on making critical decisions, such as determining which drugs should be on the organization's formulary, defining the best organizational strategy for managing a particular disease state, and selecting the most appropriate agent to treat a patient's medical condition. In addition, pharmacoeconomical research can help administrators and other managers to decide which services to implement within their organization. Consequently, pharmacoeconomical research provides valuable information that is used by a number of health care decision makers.

There are some important differences between pharmacoeconomical research and clinical trial studies. As compared to clinical trial research, pharmacoeconomical outcome research is concerned with evaluating the drug in the "real world." The primary role of clinical trials is to measure the *efficacy* and safety of a drug[2]; however, these studies are usually performed in very controlled, "test tube–like" environments. Clinical trials typically have strict inclusion criteria that may exclude patients who might otherwise receive the drug in general clinical practice. For instance, children and elderly patients are often not candidates for clinical trials and, for many years, women were excluded from these studies. Also, protocols for patient monitoring in clinical trials are usually more rigorous that what would ordinarily be employed. Given the relatively small sample size of most clinical trials, rare but serious adverse drug reactions may not be detected in these studies. Only after a drug has been used in a much larger patient population do we obtain a more accurate understanding of its safety and effectiveness, which explains why postmarketing surveillance is so important.

In contrast to clinical research, pharmacoeconomical research attempts to measure the *efficiency* of a drug or its overall value in the health care system.[3] It not only evaluates drug therapy outcomes but also compares and contrasts these outcomes in terms of their costs. Most of these studies rely on both retrospective, observational data as well as clinical trial data to obtain a more realistic assessment of a drug's safety and effectiveness. By including cost in the analysis, pharmacoeconomical studies provide information that helps determine which drugs provide the most clinical benefit for the dollars spent.

Another fundamental difference between pharmacoeconomical research and clinical trial research is how the results may be extrapolated. In general, the results of a well-designed clinical study conducted in one country are also applicable to other countries. With clinical studies, one is less concerned about where the study was conducted than how it was conducted. The same cannot be said of pharmacoeconomical studies because of differences in monetary exchange rates and cultures across countries.[3] Countries may value drug costs and outcomes differently. Therefore, one should determine where the study was conducted to see if it is applicable to a given situation.

Outcomes Evaluated in Pharmacoeconomical Studies

In pharmacoeconomical research, an *outcome* is a consequence of drug therapy intervention. The primary drug therapy outcomes that pharmacoeconomical research typically evaluate are clinical outcomes, humanistic outcomes, and economic outcomes.[1] *Clinical outcomes* include the results of treatment with a drug and may be both favorable and unfavorable. For example, a drug may cure, prevent, or slow the progression of a disease (a favorable outcome) but also have serious side effects or toxicity associated with it (an unfavorable outcome). Therefore, when pharmacoeconomical studies develop clinical outcome measures, investigators must consider all potential consequences of a therapy, not just the benefits.

In contrast to clinical outcomes, *humanistic outcomes* look at a therapy from the patients' points of view. These outcomes address such questions as how the patient feels and what they perceive their quality of life to be. A drug that prolongs a patient's life may not be considered beneficial by the patient if he or she believes quality of life has become suboptimal. For instance, a patient with a catastrophic illness may not value a drug that prolongs his or her life in the same way that a patient with a less serious medical problem would. Therefore, humanistic outcomes are very important in assessing the overall value of a medication.

Economic outcomes are the *costs* associated with a therapy. Several different types of costs are measured in pharmacoeconomical research. The first type of costs are *direct costs*, which may be both medical and nonmedical. Direct medical costs are associated with the drug and the medical care itself and would include acquisition costs, monitoring costs, preparation costs, and physicians' fees. Direct medical costs also include the cost of administrating the medication (e.g., intravenous administration sets, infusion pumps) as well as the cost of treating an adverse drug reaction. Direct nonmedical costs are those that are relevant to providing the therapy and include transportation to a health care facility and ancillary support, such as social services and home care services.[4]

Indirect costs result from loss of productivity (e.g., loss of income, days of school missed) due to illness. These are costs associated with the morbidity and mortality of a disease. Although these costs are not universally accepted as being important, they may significantly affect the total cost of a disease.[4] For example, the cost associated with loss of productivity associated with asthma is estimated to be millions of dollars.[5]

Intangible costs are more difficult to assign a dollar value. These are costs associated with pain and suffering of disease and may greatly affect a patient's well-being and quality of life. How does one put a specific dollar amount on pain and suffering (unless one is a lawyer)? Some pharmacoeconomical studies use survey instruments to assess quality of life to measure these important costs in a nonmonetary way.[4] These types of studies are discussed later in this chapter.

In reviewing the pharmacoeconomical literature, one should carefully evaluate the costs used in conducting studies to make sure that all appropriate costs have been included. Failure to consider this information may lead to inaccurate conclusions. For example, the costs associated with the preparation and administration of an intravenous drug should be included when comparing it to an oral agent. In addition, one should also determine whether the costs cited are relevant to the organization. Many pharmacoeconomical studies use average wholesale price (AWP) when comparing therapies; however, if the cost to the organization differs significantly from the AWP, then the study results may not be relevant.

Discounting Costs

Many economic studies evaluate costs and benefits at different times. For instance, a therapy may be intended to prevent a serious complication of a disease, such as stroke, and the outcome may not be realized for several years after the therapy is started. Consequently, economists believe these costs should be adjusted, or "discounted," back to their present value.

The rationale for *discounting* is that the value of the dollar today is worth more than its value would be in the future.[2] Given money now, one could invest it or realize an immediate benefit from it (e.g., spend it on a need) that would increase its value. If costs are not discounted, the benefit or cost in the first year will remain stable and may lead to a false conclusion about the value of the benefit. Although there is no generally accepted consensus about how to discount or how much to discount, the discount rate used in most studies is often between 5% and 10%. If measured in monetary units, the benefits of the therapy (e.g., cost of hospitalization avoided) should be discounted as well.

The following formula is generally used to discount a cost back to its present value:

$$(PV): PV = FC \times DF,$$

where FC is equal to the future cost, and DF is the discount factor.[6]

The discount factor is equal to $1/(1 + r)^n$, where r is the discount rate, and n is the year the cost was incurred. Therefore, the formula may be rearranged to be—

$$PV = FC \times \frac{1}{(1 + r)^n}$$

Table 9-1 illustrates what the discount factor is at a rate of 5% for years 1 through 5.

The following represents an example of how discounting is used. Suppose a therapy is projected to cost $5000 in year 1, $4000 in year 2, and $3000 in year 3. The unadjusted cost during these 3 years is $12,000 ($5000 + $4000 + $3000). However, if the costs are discounted to the present value, then the cost would be—

($5000 × 0.952) + ($4000 × 0.907) + ($3000 × 0.864), or $10,980.

The assumption made here is that expenses are realized at the end of each year; therefore, the first year's costs are discounted. An equally reasonable assumption is that expenses are incurred at the beginning of the year, in which case only the second and third year's costs would be discounted as follows:

($5000) + ($4000 × 0.952) + ($3000 × 0.907) = $11,529.[6]

Consequently, the discounted cost is dependent on both the discount rate used and interpretation of when expenses are incurred. To determine whether the results of a pharmacoeconomical study are altered by a change in either of these

TABLE 9-1. Discount Factor at 5% Rate

Year (n)	Discount Factor $(1/(1 + r)^n)$
1	0.952
2	0.907
3	0.864
4	0.823
5	0.784

variables, a sensitivity analysis should be performed. A discussion of a sensitivity analysis is provided later in this chapter.

There is some controversy regarding discounting because the discount rate used is arbitrary (e.g. 5%, 10%).[2] In addition, it is difficult to assign a discount rate to nonmonetary benefits, such as years of life saved. However, discounting does provide for a more fair comparison of alternatives if costs and benefits are realized at different times. Typically, costs are incurred in the present, and benefits are realized at some point in the future.

Perspective of a Pharmacoeconomical Study

The *perspective* of a pharmacoeconomical study is the point of view from which it is conducted. A study may be performed from the perspective of a hospital or another health care provider, a payer, a patient, or society in general. It is important to understand the study perspective because it determines which outcomes and costs will be measured.[2] For example, a pharmacoeconomical study evaluating the impact of a drug on length of stay conducted from a hospital perspective would be concerned primarily with direct costs to the institution and days of hospitalization. If the same drug were being evaluated from a societal perspective, indirect and intangible costs may be relevant. Benefits such as reduction in clinic or emergency room visits may also be measured. In contrast, the patients' perspective would focus primarily on out-of-pocket expenses and not on the overall cost of therapy. Consequently, the study perspective directs and limits how the results are interpreted and applied. Therefore, in assessing any pharmacoeconomical study, one should first determine from which perspective the study is conducted.

Pharmacoeconomical Study Designs

There are four common types of pharmacoeconomical studies. Each of these studies measures costs in dollars, but there are differences in how the outcomes are valued. An understanding of these various types of studies is important for most appropriate interpretation of the results.

Cost Minimization Analysis

The first type of pharmacoeconomical study is a *cost-minimization analysis* (CMA), which is the most basic of the research methodologies. A CMA simply compares the cost of two or more alternatives, assuming equal outcomes of each alternative. In general, the least costly alternative is selected.

For example, suppose an investigator wants to evaluate two antibiotics of the same class for the treatment of community-acquired pneumonia (CAP). Based on documentation in the literature, both are assumed to be equal in terms of outcomes. A CMA could be performed, as noted in Table 9-2. Based on this CMA analysis, antibiotic B would be the preferred agent because it costs approximately half as much as antibiotic A per day of therapy.

TABLE 9-2. **Cost Minimization Analysis**

Cost/Day ($)	Antibiotic A	Antibiotic B
Drug	30.00	10.00
Supply	5.00	2.50
Labor	5.00	2.00
Monitoring	10.00	10.00
Total	50.00	24.50

However, as stated previously, this type of methodology requires that the outcomes of the alternatives being evaluated *are identical in all respects,* which is often very difficult to demonstrate. For this particular CMA to be valid, the duration of treatment, efficacy, and toxicity all must be the same for both drugs. If they differed in any way, a CMA would not be appropriate, and another type of analysis should be performed. For example, if the incidence of a serious side effect (e.g., bone marrow suppression) were higher with antibiotic B than antibiotic A, then the cost of therapy might be higher than that predicted by the CMA. Consequently, because of the requirement that the alternatives be equal in all respects and because this is rarely the case, a CMA is not commonly used to compare drug therapies. However, a CMA can be used when equality between two alternatives can be more easily established (e.g., generic versus brand name; once a day versus multiple daily dosing of the same agent).[7]

Cost–Benefit Analysis

In contrast to a CMA, in a *cost–benefit analysis* (CBA), the outcomes of the alternatives being studied are not considered to be equal. In a CBA, both the costs and the outcomes (benefits) of the alternatives are measured in monetary units. A benefit-to-cost (B/C) ratio is then calculated to determine which alternative provides the greatest benefit relative to cost, or "most bang for the buck." If the B/C is greater than 1, then the benefits exceed the costs and the alternative is favorably received. In contrast, if the B/C ratio is less than 1, then the benefits are less than the costs and the alternative is rejected. If the B/C ratio equals 1, then a decision may need to be based on other factors (e.g., feasibility, preference). A CBA may be conducted when resources are limited and choices must be made concerning the most appropriate alternative on which to expend those resources.

One of the difficulties with this type of study is assessing a dollar value on clinical outcomes.[2] For instance, how may dollars is a year of life gained or a life saved worth? This type of study design is more useful in conducting an economical

TABLE 9-3. **Cost–Benefit Analysis**

Costs	$	Benefits	$
Salaries, including clerical support	90,000	Reduction in length of stay	250,000 (1 day/patient × 500 patients × $500/day)
Office supplies, including software	10,000	Fewer days of IV therapy, including IV supplies	50,000 (2 days/patient × 500 patients × $50/day)
Total	100,000		300,000

analysis of health care services than of therapies. For example, suppose an investigator is interested in determining whether a pharmacokinetic monitoring service is economically beneficial to an organization. One year after the service was implemented, a CBA was performed, and an analysis of the costs and benefits of the service over the first year is described in Table 9-3.

The net benefit of the pharmacokinetic service is the difference in benefits received ($300,000) and organizational costs ($100,000), or $200,000. The B/C ratio is $300,000/$100,000, or 3:1. Therefore, during the first year of operation, the organization saved $3 for every $1 spent on the service.

However, suppose no change in length of stay was noted over the first year and the only benefits reported were a reduction in intravenous (IV) therapy costs. The B/C ratio would be $50,000/$100,000 or 1:2. In this scenario, the pharmacokinetic service would be considered to cost more than it is worth (e.g., a $1 return on each $2 invested).

Whereas a CBA is of limited value in comparing drug therapies, it can be a useful tool that administrative decision makers can use for evaluating the value of existing services as well as projecting the potential benefits of proposed services.

Cost-Effectiveness Analysis

In a *cost-effectiveness analysis* (CEA), the outcomes of the alternatives are not measured in monetary units, but rather in natural or physical units (e.g., years of life saved, complication avoided). Although a CEA does not assume equal outcomes, it should compare alternatives with similar objectives (e.g., prevention or treatment of same disease). A CEA is primarily used when decisions concerning the relative costs and benefits of alternative therapies are not apparent.

Table 9-4 illustrates the various ways that the cost-effectiveness of alternative therapies may be interpreted based on their costs and outcomes. As noted in the table, when the costs of an alternative are high and the efficacy is low, or when the

TABLE 9-4. Interpreting Cost-Effectiveness

	COST	
	Higher Cost	Lower Cost
OUTCOME		
Higher effectivenes	May be cost-effective	Cost-effective
Lower effectiveness	Not cost-effective	May be cost-effective

costs are low and the efficacy is high, cost-effectiveness decisions are fairly obvious. However, when a therapy may be both less expensive and less effective than the alternative, or more expensive and more effective, the relative cost-effectiveness must be established to determine whether any additional benefit is worth the extra cost. A drug that is cost-effective does not mean it is the least costly or the most effective. It simply reflects the added value of the drug relative to alternatives. For example, suppose one wants to determine which antibiotic, A or B, to use for primary treatment of CAP, as described earlier in the discussion of CMA. However, because of differences in efficacy and adverse reactions between the two drugs, a CMA would not be valid; therefore, one has to perform a different type of study. Because it is difficult to put a dollar cost on clinical outcomes, a CEA would be more appropriate than a CBA.

Many CEAs are preformed by decision analysis. A decision analysis model, or "tree," is created that plots all possible outcomes, the probability of each of those outcomes occurring, and the potential costs associated with each of the outcomes. The information for these decision trees may be based on either published information or one's own outcome research. If the information is obtained from information from the primary literature, then the nature of the data (e.g., randomized, controlled clinical trial, observational study) should be evaluated to assess their validity.

Figure 9-1 illustrates a very simple decision tree for the antibiotic comparison example. Both positive (treatment success) and negative (treatment failure, adverse drug reaction) outcomes should be included in the analysis, as should the costs associated with each. Most decision trees are far more complex than this one and include many more possible outcomes (e.g., specific type of adverse drug reaction, whether hospitalization was required). One can then calculate the cost of an outcome based on the *cumulative probability* of the path selected. For example, a patient treated with antibiotic A has a probability for success of 0.90. The probability that the patient will experience an adverse drug reaction during a successful course of therapy is 0.15. Therefore, the cumulative probability of following path 2 is (0.90×0.15), or 0.14. This is then multiplied by the cost of that outcome ($1200). An analysis of different outcomes, cumulative probabilities and costs for both antibiotics, is summarized in Table 9-5.

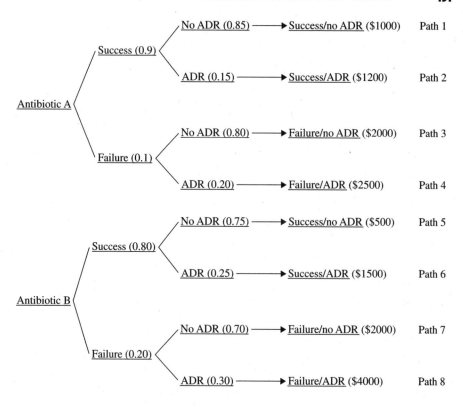

Figure 9-1. Decision tree for antibiotic therapies A and B.
(ADR = adverse drug reaction.)

One can now determine a cost-effectiveness (C/E) ratio. The C/E for each antibiotic is the total cost of all treatment outcomes divided by the overall success rate. Thus, for antibiotic A, the C/E ratio is $1137 ÷ 0.90, or $1263, per treated patient. For antibiotic B, the C/E ratio is $1120 ÷ 0.80, or $1400, per treated patient. Based on this analysis, antibiotic A would be considered more cost-effective than antibiotic B. Although antibiotic B may be less expensive than antibiotic A, the probability of treatment success is less, and it has a higher probability of adverse reactions associated with it. Therefore, by taking in account all possible outcomes and their probability of occurring, this type of analysis can evaluate the relative cost-effectiveness of alternatives. Again, one should be careful not to interpret cost-effectiveness as being more effective or less costly. As noted previously, this analysis is useful when outcomes in efficacy and costs between alternatives differ and one is uncertain about the benefits of added costs.

Sensitivity Analysis. The CEA evaluating antibiotics A and B is based on assuming that outcomes will occur at a defined frequency; however, these assumptions do

TABLE 9-5. Cost of Antibiotic Therapy Based on Outcomes

Outcome	Average Cost ($)	Cumulative Probability	Cost of Path ($)
		Antibiotic A	
Cure, no ADR	1000	0.76	765
Cure, ADR	1200	0.14	162
Failure, no ADR	2000	0.08	160
Failure, ADR	2500	0.02	50
Total cost			1137
		Antibiotic B	
Cure, no ADR	500	0.60	300
Cure, ADR	1500	0.20	300
Failure, no ADR	2000	0.14	280
Failure, ADR	4000	0.06	240
Total cost			1120

Note: ADR = adverse drug reaction.

not take into account variances in the probability of any event occurring. For example, suppose the probability of an adverse drug reaction during a successful course of treatment with antibiotic A was 0.2 instead of 0.15. Alternatively, what if the success rate with antibiotic B were 0.85 and not 0.80? In addition, drug costs may differ, which may also affect the results of a CEA.

Because the probability of an outcome may differ from that used in a decision tree analysis, a *sensitivity analysis* should be conducted to validate the results. A sensitivity analysis is based on creating a number of "what-if" scenarios to determine whether the results of the study are valid only under certain assumptions.[8] For example, a drug may be considered to be cost-effective only at a particularly low dose and only if the probability for success exceeds a certain value. Therefore, a sensitivity analysis assigns different costs and probabilities for outcomes to learn whether the results hold true under a variety of reasonable possibilities. For more complex decision trees, a Monte-Carlo simulation can be performed. This common technique randomly assigns different values and recalculates outcomes based on a number of hypothetical situations.

Incremental Cost-Effectiveness Analysis. As described previously, a CEA analysis expresses an average C/E ratio for the alternatives being compared. However, one may be interested in learning whether the additional cost of a more expensive therapy or program would provide added value. Rather than just comparing average C/E ratios, one may want to assess cost differences between one alternative and the next least or most effective option. This information may be helpful in prioritizing various alternatives, especially in developing disease-state management programs.

To determine cost differences between therapeutic alternatives, an *incremental cost-effectiveness analysis* (ICA) should be performed. An ICA represents the additional cost and effectiveness gained when two or more alternatives are compared. An ICA assesses the *added cost per net effect* for the alternative therapy and is the difference in total costs (C) of two therapies divided by difference in *effectiveness* (E) of the two therapies[8]:

$$((C_2 - C_1) \div (E_2 - E_1))$$

For example, if therapy A costs \$50,000 and saves 10 lives, it has an average cost-effectiveness (C/E) ratio of \$50,000 ÷ 10, or \$5000/life saved. If therapy B costs \$90,000 and saves 15 lives, it has an average C/E ratio of \$90,000 ÷ 15, or \$6000/life saved. However, the ICA for therapy B would be equal to the difference in cost of therapies divided by the difference in effectiveness or (\$90,000 − \$50,000 ÷ (15 − 10), or \$8000/life saved. Consequently, by using only the average cost-effectiveness ratio to evaluate therapy B as compared with therapy A, one may actually underestimate the additional cost per life saved.[8] Therefore, when comparing therapies or services, an ICA provides a better analysis of the extra value gained per dollars spent.

Cost–Utility Analysis

A cost–utility analysis (CUA) is similar to a CEA, but the measured outcomes take into account patient health preferences, or "utilities." Outcomes are measured as quality-adjusted life years (QALYs), which considers the fact that not each year of life gained from a therapy is valued by a patient equally. For example, a patient with a debilitating disease (e.g., cancer) may not perceive a year of life saved in the same way as an otherwise healthy patient with a very manageable condition, such as hypertension. Patients may express their preferences on a rating scale of 1 (perfect health) to 0 (dead).[7] For instance, a disease that reduces a patient's quality of life by 50%, will take away 0.5 QALYs per year.

As an example of how a CUA can be important in determining cost-effectiveness, assume that a drug has a C/E ratio of \$500 per year of life gained. However, suppose a patient rates that year of life gained as only 0.5 on a scale of 0 through 1. When adjusting for QALYs, the cost of the therapy now would be \$1000 per year of life gained (\$500 ÷ 0.5). Therefore, a treatment that adds 1 year of good health is preferable to that which adds 1 year of poor health.

One of the limitations of a CUA is that there is no universally accepted method for measuring patient utilities. However, authors of CUA studies should indicate which method they used and whether it has been validated as an appropriate assessment instrument. This type of analysis is more difficult to perform than the others described previously and is less frequently reported in the literature.

However, a CUA may be important in comparing therapies when quality of life is an important consideration (e.g., antineoplastic agents).

Conclusion

Pharmacoeconomical research plays an increasingly important role in making critical decisions concerning options regarding drug therapies and pharmaceutical services. Pharmacists should have a basic understanding of pharmacoeconomical concepts and the research methods employed to most effectively use the information gained from this rapidly growing field.

References

1. Reeder CE. Overview of pharmacoeconomics and pharmaceutical outcome evaluations. Am J Health-Sys Pharm. 1995;52 (Suppl 4):S5–S8.

2. Johnson JA, Coons SJ. Evaluation of published pharmacoeconomic studies. J Pharm Pract. 1995;8:156–166.

3. Milne RJ. Evaluation of the pharmacoeconomic literature. *Pharmacoeconomics.* 1994;6:337–345.

4. Sacristan JA, Soto J, Galende I. Evaluation of pharmacoeconomic studies: utilization of a checklist. *Ann Pharmacotherapy.* 1993;27:1126–1233.

5. National Asthma Education and Prevention Program Task Force. Report on cost-effectiveness, quality of care, and financing of asthma care. *Am J Resp Crit Care Med.* 1996;154(Suppl 1);S81–S130.

6. Bootman, JL, Townsend RJ, McGhan WF. *Principles of Pharmacoeconomics.* Cincinnati, Ohio: Harvey Whitney Books; 1991.

7. Jolicoeur LM, Jones-Grizzle AJ, Boyer JG. Guidelines for performing a pharmacoeconomic analysis. Am J Hosp Pharm. 1992;49:1741–1747.

8. Udvarhelyi IS, Colditz GA, Arti Ri AB, et al. Cost-effectiveness and cost-benefit analyses in the medical literature. *Ann Intern Med.* 1992;116:238–244.

Study Questions

1. Define pharmacoeconomics.

2. Describe two ways in which a pharmacoeconomical study differs from clinical trial.

3. Define the following terms used in pharmacoeconomic studies:

    a. Clinical outcomes

    b. Humanistic outcomes

    c. Direct medical costs

    d. Direct nonmedical costs

    e. Indirect costs

TABLE 9-6. Pharmacy Director's Data

Costs	With Clinic ($)	Before Clinic ($)
Costs of clinic visits	2000	500
Trips to emergency room	800	2400
Hospitalizations	50,000	175,000
Salary and benefits	80,000	000
Total	132,800	177,900

    f. Intangible costs

    g. Discounting

    h. Study perspective

4. For a cost-minimization analysis to be valid, what major assumption must be met?

5. A pharmacy director needs to justify continued funding beyond the first year of operation for a pharmacist-based anticoagulation clinic. To provide support for the service, the director conducts a cost–benefit analysis. The director compares the costs of the clinic to that of the previous year with no clinic. Table 9-6 summarizes the director's data.

    a. What would be the benefit-to-cost ratio of the anticoagulation clinic?

    b. Based on the benefit-to-cost ratio calculated, is the anticoagulation clinic cost-beneficial? Describe what this ratio means.

6. You are trying to determine whether a new drug (drug A) is more cost-effective for the treatment of peptic ulcer disease than an existing formulary agent (drug B). Based on your organization's experience and published outcome data, you construct the decision tree displayed in Figure 9-2.

    a. Based on the probabilities and costs cited, what is the average cost-effectiveness (C/E) ratio of drug A?

    b. Based on the probabilities and costs cited, what is the average C/E ratio of drug B?

    c. Which agent would be considered the more cost-effective?

7. You find information supporting a higher success rate for drug B in Question 6. If the success rate for drug B is assumed to be 80% instead of 65%, would your conclusion as to the most cost-effective agent be different?

8. Therapy A has a cost of $1800/course of therapy and a treatment success rate of 70%. Therapy B has a cost of $2000/course of therapy and a treatment success rate of 90%. What is the incremental cost-effectiveness of treatment B as compared to treatment A?

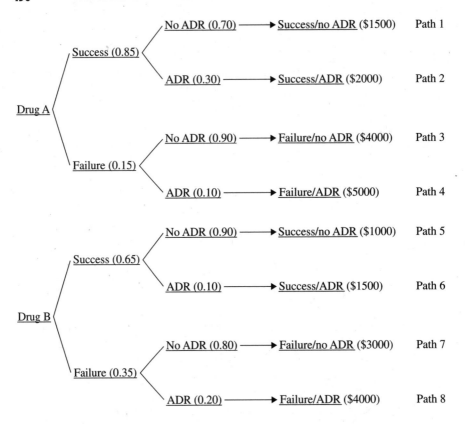

Figure 9-2. Decision tree for cost-effectiveness analysis.
(ADR = adverse drug reaction.)

9. Table 9-7 describes the outcomes of two drug treatments for the treatment of chronic obstructive pulmonary disease.

    a. How many QALYs are gained with therapy A?

    b. How many QALYs are gained with therapy B?

    c. What is the incremental cost–utility of therapy A?

TABLE 9-7. Outcomes of Two Drug Treatments for COPD

Drug	Cost ($)	Life Expectancy (years)	Quality of Life
Drug A	50,000	6	0.80
Drug B	15,000	5	0.90

10. Table 9-8 describes the costs and benefits estimated for a new drug to reduce cardiovascular complications during the first 5 years per 100 patients treated.

a. What is the B/C ratio?

b. Using a discount rate of 5% (see Table 9-1), now calculate the B/C ratio. (Assume costs incurred at year end.)

c. Explain how discounting would change your interpretation of the cost–benefit of this drug.

TABLE 9-8. Estimated Costs and Benefits for a New Drug

Year	Costs ($)	Benefits ($)
1	50,000	10,000
2	50,000	10,000
3	20,000	40,000
4	20,000	50,000
5	10,000	50,000

Pharmacoepidemiology in Pharmacy Practice

Pharmacoepidemiological concepts and methods are frequently applied in pharmacy practice. Perhaps the most common application of pharmacoepidemiology is the use of information obtained from pharmacoepidemiological studies to make drug therapy decisions. The best clinical decisions are based on solid evidence. This chapter discusses the incorporation of evidence-based medicine into clinical practice.

Other areas to which pharmacists apply pharmacoepidemiological methods include adverse drug reaction surveillance, drug utilization evaluations (DUEs), and pharmacoeconomical analyses. All of these functions provide pharmacists with excellent sources of data to conduct more formalized pharmacoepidemiological research. This chapter also discusses how to apply the pharmacoepidemiological methods discussed throughout this book to the practice of pharmacy. Resources available to pharmacists who wish to practice in the area of pharmacoepidemiology are discussed as well.

Evidence-Based Medicine

The best drug therapy decisions are decisions based on sound evidence. Evidence that a drug is safe and effective is obtained from pharmacoepidemiological studies and disseminated via the medical literature. Medical literature can be classified as primary, secondary, or tertiary.

Primary medical literature provides new information to the field of medicine and consists of descriptive, observational, and interventional studies. All of these study designs are used to provide new information about the use or effect of a particular drug in a specific population. These studies are then published in pharmacy and medical journals.

Hundreds of medical journals are published every week. These journals fall into either general or specialty categories. General medical journals publish information on topics of interest to general practitioners, whereas specialty medical journals publish in specific areas of medical practice (e.g., dermatology, cardiology). To remain current in the field of practice, practitioners typically subscribe to a few medical journals within their scope of practice.

Secondary medical literature consists of indexing systems. It is impractical to search one by one through the thousands of editions of medical journals to find clinical information. The secondary systems allow practitioners to search through the vast array of medical journals to find information about a particular subject. Search terms are entered into a database, and the database then reveals when and where information has been published on the topic of interest. Some databases provide access to complete article(s), and others provide information only on where to locate the article(s). The most commonly used indexing system is the Medline database, which was created in 1966 and indexes more than 1600 medical journals.

Tertiary medical literature consists of literature reviews, which can be in the form of textbooks, reference books, or review articles in medical journals. Before a review is written, a literature search is conducted using the secondary systems to identify all of the articles published on a particular subject. The information is then collated and presented in a manner that is easily used by practitioners. Tertiary resources are quick, efficient resources that are used to answer questions about the most common clinical problems.

Clinicians use all types of literature in the course of caring for patients. Suppose a patient presents to a clinician complaining of a racing heartbeat (i.e., tachycardia). The clinician conducts a complete medical history and physical examination of the patient. All factors must be considered before determining the cause of the tachycardia. If the clinician suspects the tachycardia is an adverse drug reaction associated with a particular medication, then he or she attempts to find evidence in the literature that supports the suspicion. As stated previously, the best clinical decisions are based on sound medical evidence, rather than hunches or suspicions.

To obtain medical evidence on a particular topic, clinicians first searches the tertiary literature (e.g., textbooks, reference books). If no information is found, a literature search using the secondary systems is conducted. A literature search reveals where and when information on the topic has been published, and the clinician must then retrieve and review all of the articles. The studies must be critiqued with regard to design, methodology, quality of data, and bias. A clinical decision based on sound evidence is then made that either supports or negates the theory that the tachycardia is associated with the use of the drug.

Archie Cochrane, a physician-epidemiologist, realized that conducting exhaustive literature searches and medical literature reviews were daunting and time-consuming tasks requiring many resources.[1] Clinicians do not have the time or the resources required to conduct such searches on every clinical situation they encounter during the course of a day. Cochrane believed that clinicians should be able to conduct a search on a specific topic and find a well-conducted, systematic review that identifies and summarizes all of the medical literature published on a particular topic.[1] He enlisted a group of international collaborators to create and maintain such a database; it is called the Cochrane Database of Systematic Reviews.[1]

The Cochrane collaborators attempt to provide accurate, unbiased systematic reviews to be used specifically for clinical decision making. [1] Cochrane reviews are conducted for both traditional and complementary medicine. They have included reviews on herbal medicine, homeopathy, acupuncture, and massage.[2] Cochrane collaborators perform exhaustive searches for published and unpublished studies in English and other languages.[1] Whenever possible, the Cochrane reviews are based on randomized clinical trials, which are considered the gold standard in medical research. If randomized clinical trials are not available, then the strongest observational studies—the best designed and conducted studies—are used in the Cochrane reviews.[1] After completion, the reviews undergo rigorous peer review. Whereas a meta-analysis is conducted and appears once in a journal, Cochrane reviews are updated on a regular basis to include new information.[1]

Jaded et al. conducted a study to compare the quality of meta-analyses published in medical journals with the quality of the Cochrane reviews.[3] Twelve Cochrane reviews on the treatment of asthma were compared to 38 meta-analyses published in 22 peer-reviewed journals. Jaded and colleagues concluded that most of the meta-analyses published in peer-reviewed journals had a significant number of methodological flaws that limited their utility; the Cochrane reviews were determined to be of better quality than the published meta-analyses.[3]

Adverse Drug Reaction Surveillance

Adverse drug reaction reporting and monitoring plays an important role in the postmarketing surveillance of drugs. As mentioned in Chapter 6, pharmacists play an integral part in adverse drug reaction reporting. In fact, historically, pharmacists have the highest rate of adverse drug reaction reporting among health care professionals.

The routine collection of adverse drug reactions in a health care system provides a valuable source of data for pharmacists to use in the conduct of pharmacoepidemiological research. Typically, pharmacists collect and report adverse drug reactions on a regular basis to pharmacy and therapeutics committees (P&T committees). These reports are most commonly used to monitor the safety of drugs within institutions, but pharmacists are usually also responsible for forwarding serious adverse drug reactions to the Food and Drug Administration (FDA). Just as the FDA acts after receiving several serious adverse drug reactions associated with a particular drug, the P&T committees of individual institutions react to serious adverse drug reactions within the institution by creating medication guidelines and restrictions.

The limitations of spontaneous adverse drug reaction reports should be considered before action is taken to restrict the use of a drug. Confounding information is often incomplete or inaccurate in adverse drug reaction reports, which is why it becomes difficult to determine the causality of the reaction in critically ill patients taking several medications. Spontaneous reports are subject to observation bias, and other limitations include inadequate information on the total number of patients exposed to the drug and the absence of a control group for comparison.

Adverse drug reactions are often confused with medical errors in a surveillance system. It is equally important to monitor prescribers in a surveillance system to determine the causality of the medication problem. Some practitioners may be prescribing the drug inappropriately, with regard to indication, dose, length of therapy, and so forth. The information presumed and reported as an adverse drug reaction may actually be a prescribing error.

Rather than using adverse drug reaction reports to create medication guidelines and restrictions, pharmacists may instead choose to study a particular drug reaction further using pharmacoepidemiological methods. For example, a cohort study could be conducted comparing subjects exposed to the drug with subjects not exposed to the drug for development of the adverse drug reaction. A case-control study could also be conducted to compare subjects who experienced the adverse drug reaction, to subjects who did not, for exposure to the particular drug. Information can be collected on person, place, and time related to the drug exposure. Data on both prescribers and users can be collected and analyzed.

The benefits of using more formal pharmacoepidemiological methods include the ability to quantify the rate at which the adverse drug reaction is occurring and the ability to identify various risk factors associated with it. The results of these observational studies can then be used to create guidelines and restrictions on the use of drugs within institutions.

Drug Utilization Studies

The World Health Organization (WHO) defines drug utilization as "the marketing, distribution, prescription, and use of drugs in a society, with special emphasis on the resulting medical, social, and economic consequences."[4] Pharmacists conduct drug utilization studies, or DUEs, as part of their routine activities. Like adverse drug reaction monitoring, the Joint Commission for the Accreditation of Health Care Organizations (JCAHO) requires health care institutions to conduct drug utilization studies.

DUEs are most commonly conducted to monitor prescribing patterns. Medications monitored via DUE are chosen according to cost, frequency of use, and risk of toxicity. Whereas cost and frequency of use are easily obtained, the risk of toxicity is typically unknown at the time the DUE is designed and originated. Drugs newly approved by the FDA that have shown serious adverse effects in phase III trials are typically chosen to be monitored via DUEs.

For example, when alteplase (TPA®) was first approved by the FDA, many practitioners were concerned about the bleeding side effects that had occurred in phase III trials. Consequently, pharmacists chose to conduct DUEs to monitor the use of alteplase. Information was collected on both prescribers and patients. Data collected on patients included demographic information, past medical history, indication, dose, duration of therapy, and specific documentation of unintended bleeding effects. The goal of the DUEs was to monitor the use of alteplase to ensure that the drug was being used as indicated in the proper patients and to measure the extent of bleeding associated with alteplase.

DUEs are similar to cohort studies. Subjects exposed to a particular drug are followed for a period to determine the incidence of an adverse reaction. These DUEs can easily be expanded to a prospective cohort model. By collecting information on similar subjects not exposed to the drug of interest, the pharmacist can better estimate the relationship between the adverse event and the drug.

Pharmacoepidemiological methods can also be used to determine other "problem" drugs to monitor via DUEs. As mentioned previously with regard to adverse drug reaction monitoring, observational studies can be used to identify serious ADRs or prescribing errors.

Pharmacoeconomics

As discussed in Chapter 9, pharmacoeconomical analyses are used to determine the value of drug therapies. Such analyses assess various types of outcomes, including economic, clinical, and humanistic ones.[5]

Pharmacoeconomical analyses can be used in formulary decision making.[6] Numerous P&T committees have already incorporated pharmacoeconomical analyses into formulary management activities. These methods can be used to determine which drugs should be added to the formulary, but these methods are also helpful in evaluating the value of drugs after the institution has some experience using the medications.

Pharmacoeconomical analyses can also be used in disease-state management.[7] Disease-state management involves the creation of clinical guidelines for diagnosis and treatment. Decisions regarding which drugs to include in treatment guidelines can be made using pharmacoeconomical analyses.

Pharmacoepidemiological Research as an Extension of Daily Clinical Practice

Pharmacists in clinical settings monitor the uses and effects of drugs on a daily basis. Clinical pharmacists collect information about individual patients; however, pharmacists can also choose to view patients as populations, rather than individuals, for the purpose of epidemiological research. If information collected about patients is systematic and routine, then the routine monitoring of individual patients can easily be applied to a cohort study design. The data collected can then be analyzed to generate new hypotheses or to identify trends of drug use.

For example, a pharmacist conducting rounds in a critical care unit will collect information about individual patients with regard to demographics, past medical history, current medical problems, laboratory data, physical findings, and so forth. The pharmacist will monitor each individual patient in an effort to optimize pharmaceutical care. The data collection may or may not be consistent from patient to patient. In this scenario, the information is typically used solely for the purpose of caring for the patient.

The pharmacist could instead choose to develop data-collection forms to be used on all patients. If data collection is systematic and consistent, then the data can be analyzed to determine the effects of drugs within populations of patients, rather than thinking of patients only as individuals. New hypotheses can be generated from the data collection and analysis; these hypotheses can then be tested using more sophisticated observational or interventional studies.

Pharmacoepidemiology and Research in the Pharmacy Curriculum

There is relatively little teaching pertaining to research in pharmacy curricula. Few pharmacy schools require courses in research methodology, and even fewer require students to conduct original research.

Murphy and colleagues conducted a survey study to measure the extent of research education that doctoral students in pharmacy programs receive. Murphy reported that only 53.7% of entry-level programs required coursework in research methodology, and even fewer require students to conduct research.[8]

To actively participate in pharmacoepidemiological research, pharmacists need to acquire research skills. The incorporation of more research-related courses and projects into pharmacy curricula would provide the skills required to conduct quality research.

Professional Resources

Many professional resources are available to pharmacists who wish to practice or increase their knowledge in the area of pharmacoepidemiology. Several professional organizations exist in the area of epidemiology, and these organizations hold regular meetings to discuss research issues and to disseminate new findings. Many other journals are available, and pharmacists can subscribe to remain current in epidemiology. Table 10-1 lists professional organizations and professional journals pertaining to epidemiology.

The growth of the Internet has produced many Web sites dedicated to epidemiology. These sites offer information and links to professional organizations, books and journals, online courses, graduate and certificate programs, and downloadable statistical software, for example. Table 10-2 lists Web and e-mail addresses related to epidemiology.

Summary

Pharmacoepidemiology is a rapidly expanding field of practice. Pharmacists bring a unique perspective to pharmacoepidemiological research. Increased emphasis on research methods in pharmacy curricula will enable future pharmacists to participate to a greater extent in pharmacoepidemiological research and, consequently, add to the body of literature pertaining to drug use and safety.

Practicing pharmacists can apply pharmacoepidemiological methods to their practice to measure the use and effects of drugs. DUEs can be expanded to prospective cohorts for better determination of the relationships between drug exposures and desired or undesired outcomes. Adverse drug reaction surveillance

TABLE 10-1. Professional Organizations and Journals in Epidemiology

Professional organizations

American College of Epidemiology

American Public Health Association

American Statistical Association, Section on Epidemiology

Association for Professionals in Infection Control & Epidemiology

Canadian Society for Epidemiology and Biostatistics

European Society of Clinical Pharmacy

International Society for Pharmacoepidemiology

Society for Epidemiologic Research

Professional journals

American Journal of Epidemiology

American Journal of Public Health

Annals of Epidemiology

Biometrics

Drug Safety

Emerging Infectious Diseases

Epidemiologic Reviews

Epidemiology

Epidemiology and Infection

Journal of Clinical Epidemiology

Journal of Epidemiology and Community Health

MMWR: Morbidity and Mortality Weekly Report

Pharmacoepidemiology and Drug Safety

Society for Clinical Trials

Viral and Health Statistics

Weekly Epidemiological Record

World Health Statistics Quarterly

TABLE 10-2. **Web Resources Related to Epidemiology**

Type of Site	E-mail/Web Address
List serves	
Epidemiology Discussion Group	E-mail address: <u>LISTPROC@CC.UMONTREAL.CA.</u> To subscribe, include "subscribe epidemio-1 [your first and last names]" in the body of the message.
Epi Info Discussion Group	E-mail address: majordomo@mailhost.tcs.tulane.edu. To subscribe, include "subscribe epi-info end" in the body of the message.
EPIWORLD Discussion Group	E-mail address: <u>LISTSERV@UNIVSCVM.CSD.SC.EDU.</u> To subscribe, include "sub epiworld [your first and last names]" in the body of the message.
Pharmacoepidemiology & Pharmacoeconomics Discussion Group	Web address: www.egroups.com/group/pharmacoepidemiology.
Epidemiology directory	
Virtual Library-Epidemiology	www.epibiostat.ucsf.edu/epidem/epidem.html
Downloadable Statistical Software	
Epi Info	www.cdc.gov/epo/epi/epiinfo.htm

can be expanded to include not only spontaneous reports but also case-control studies using medical record review or computerized databases to quantify the relationship between drugs and adverse events. Clinical pharmacists collecting information about individual patients can systematically collect information about groups or populations of patients and then analyze the data for trends. Pharmacoeconomic analyses can be included in formulary decision making and disease-state management to determine the value of drug therapies.

References

1. Bero L, Rennie D. The Cochrane collaboration: Preparing, maintaining, and disseminating systematic reviews of the effects of health care. *JAMA.* 1995; 274(24):1935–1938.

2. *The Cochrane Library.* Issue 2. Oxford, England: Updated Software; 2000.

3. Jadad AR, Moher M, Browman GP, et al. Systematic reviews and meta-analyses of asthma:critical evaluation. *BMJ.* 2000;320:537–540.

4. World Health Organization Expert Committee. *The Selection of Essential Drugs.* Technical Report Series No. 615. Geneva, World Health Organization, 1977.

5. Kozma CM, Reeder CE, Schulz RM. Economic, clinical, and humanistic outcomes: A planning model for pharmacoeconomic research. *Clin Ther.* 1993; 15(6):1121–1132.

6. Sanchez LA. Pharmacoeconomics and formulary decision making. *Pharmacoeconomics.* 1996;9(Suppl. 1):16–25.

7. Thomas N. The role of pharmacoeconomics in disease management. *Pharmacoeconomics.* 1996;9(Suppl. 1):9–15.

8. Murphy JE, Peralta LS, Kirking DM. Research experiences and research-related coursework in the education of doctors of pharmacy. *Pharmacotherapy.* 1999; 19(2):213–220.

Study Questions

1. Describe how evidence-based medicine is used to make therapeutic decisions.

2. What PMS methods can be applied to institutional adverse drug reaction reporting systems?

3. What PMS methods can be applied to DUEs?

4. How can pharmacoeconomical methods be applied to pharmacy practice?

5. How can a practicing pharmacist incorporate pharmacoepidemiological investigations into daily work?

Answer Key for Study Questions

Chapter 1

1. The primary difference in the focus of inquiry between clinical medicine and epidemiology involves the emphasis on the individual patient versus the population at large. Clinical medicine focuses on individual patients and may not be able to differentiate variability between patients, whereas epidemiology focuses on large groups of people or populations and what happens to whole groups.

2. The first "clinical drug trial" was performed by James Lind from 1747 through 1753. Lind performed a study on sailors aboard a ship at sea. He tested 6 treatments or interventions for scurvy by using 6 pairs of sailors (thus, 6 different treatment groups). Two sailors received citrus fruit and showed the greatest improvement.

3. In the host–agent–environment model, the host is the recipient of the disease. Host factors, also referred to as intrinsic factors, refer to various demographic as well as behavioral aspects of the host, human beings. The agent of disease, also called an etiological factor, can consist of a variety of things that are related to or cause specific disease states. The environment, or extrinsic factors, consists of the physical and social setting in which the host and agent interact, possibly leading to disease.

4. Definitions

a. *Onset* of a disease outbreak is represented by the first case exhibiting the signs and symptoms of that disease.

b. *Etiology* refers to the causative agent or risk factor that produces disease.

c. A *vehicle* is an inanimate object that may aid in the transmission, or spread, of a causative agent of disease.

d. A *vector* is an animate or living thing that may aid in the transmission, or spread, of a causative agent of disease.

e. *Portals of entry or exit* are the ways in which the causative agent enters and leaves the host.

f. A *reservoir* is a place where the causative agent may reside or spend part of its life cycle.

g. *Mode of transmission* refers to the ways in which a causative agent or risk factor may spread throughout a population.

h. An *epidemic*, also called an outbreak, is a sudden, dramatic increase in the number of people with a specific disease or problem. It is usually defined in terms of a specific population in an area over a period of time.

i. An *incubation period* is the interval of time between exposure to, or contact with, the causative agent or risk factor and the onset of the symptoms or condition.

j. *Epidemiology* is the study of disease occurrence in a human population. It also considers the distribution and determinants of disease. It may also be considered the method of public health.

k. *Pharmacoepidemiology* is the study of the nature and extent of drug-taking behaviors and drug use problems. It measures the source, diffusion, use, and effects of drugs in populations, with a focus on pharmaceutical care outcomes and the identification of potential or realized drug use problems.

5. **a.** The specific denominator indicating the total number of people using Seldane® was not provided. It is, therefore, difficult to know what proportion of the population includes the hundreds of deaths from this drug.

b. A potential denominator was provided in the form of the number of prescriptions that had been filled by pharmacists. Although calculation of the proportion of people experiencing death from Seldane® use could not be based on the actual number of users, it could be calculated based on the number of prescriptions that had been dispensed. This number is much less meaningful than a number based on actual users.

c. The number of deaths, 200, divided by the number of prescriptions, 6.5 million, equals 0.0000307 deaths per prescriptions dispensed. This number is difficult to read and use in comparisons, so it can be converted to a more manageable form by multiplying it by 1 (100,000/100,000) to arrive at the number 3.07 deaths/100,000 prescriptions dispensed.

d. The number of deaths, 2000, divided by the number of prescriptions, 6.5 million, equals 0.000307, multiplied by 1 (100,000/100,000), equals 30.7 deaths/100,000 prescriptions dispensed. This number could also be expressed as 3.07 deaths/10,000 prescriptions dispensed, which can be obtained by multiplying both the numerator and the denominator by 10,000.

6. a. From an individual patient perspective, perhaps 26 deaths is sufficient reason to withdrawal the drug. But, if the drug is benefiting many other patients, then an assessment of its risks in light of its benefits must be made. For instance, if the 26 deaths occurred in 2,600,000 users of the drug, then the individual patient's risk of dying from using the drug is 1 (death)/100,000 users, or 1 in 100,000 (1:100,000), or 0.001%, compared with the beneficial effects they receive. This type of information assists clinicians in determining the best course of action for their patients.

b. Denominator data, the number of drug users or number of prescriptions, were not mentioned in the news story.

c. The number of deaths, 26, divided by the number of prescriptions, 650,000, multiplied by 1 (100,000/100,000), equals 4 deaths/100,000 prescriptions dispensed.

Chapter 2

1. The answer is c. Males have an age-adjusted mortality rate that is 70% higher than females.

2. The answer is c, an incubation period.

3. The answer is d, case fatality rate.

4. Definitions

a. *Medical surveillance* is the process of detection, performed to identify changes in the distribution of diseases so that they can be prevented or controlled within a population. Medical surveillance involves the following key features: (1) continuous data collection and evaluation, (2) an identified target population, (3) a standard definition of the outcome under study, (4) timely collection and dissemination of information, and (5) application of the data to disease control and prevention.

b. A *proportion* is a type of ratio, and a percentage is a special type of proportion. A proportion is a relation between the amount, number, size, or degree of one item and the amount, number, size, or degree of another item. A proportion is basically a ratio whose numerator is contained in its denominator.

c. A *rate* is the amount or number of one item measured in relation to units of another item. A rate is the measure (the number or frequency) of an event, condition, injury, disability, or death per unit size of a population during a specified time period. There are three basic numbers needed to develop a rate: the numerator (which consists of the number of individuals affected or ill); the denominator (the total population of a specified area under study, of which the cases in the numerator are a part or from which the cases are derived); and a specific time period.

d. *Morbidity* refers to disease, illness, injury, disorder, or sickness. Morbidity is the extent of disease, illness, injury, or disability in a defined population. It is a deviation from a state of health and well-being or the presence of a specific symptom or condition. Morbidity is usually expressed in terms of prevalence, attack rates, or incidence rates. In essence, morbidity refers to the rate of disease in a population—the number of ill people present in a certain population, which is often a healthy or at-risk group.

e. *Mortality* means death, or it describes death and related issues. The mortality rate is the rapidity with which people in a given population die of a particular condition.

f. *Prevalence* is the number of cases of a disease or condition (number of infected people) present in a defined population at one particular point in time. Prevalence also may be viewed as the probability that a condition exists in a specific population. It is the probability of occurrence of a condition, and it is sometimes called point prevalence.

g. *Period prevalence* is the probability of occurrence, or the total number of individuals with the condition or disease, during a specified period, instead of at one point in time.

h. *Incidence rate* is a measure of the rapidity with which a new condition develops in a population. It is the rate at which the condition develops or the rate at which newly diagnosed patients are identified over time.

i. *Cumulative incidence* is the probability of developing a condition within a specified period. It also can be viewed as a measure of risk. The cumulative incidence rate is useful in prospective and longitudinal studies.

j. *Incidence rate in person-time units* refers to incidence measured in person-time units due to individuals being at risk or observed for different time periods during the study. It is the sum of observation time periods during which individuals are at risk for all people in the study.

k. *Survival rate* is the likelihood of living for a specified time period after the diagnosis of a particular condition.

l. *Rate adjustment* refers to adjustments or standardizations of category-specific rates. The technique involves a procedure for overall comparison of two or more populations in which background or baseline differences in the distribution of values for a variable (e.g., underlying differences in age) are removed. It is an analytical procedure with mathematical calculations and transformations for obtaining a summary measure for a population by applying standard weights to the measures within subgroups of the population. Rate adjustments are often done to identify confounding variables.

m. *Classification* is the process of categorizing (labeling or defining) subjects in a study by a specific value (or range of values; e.g., blood pressure) or set of items (e.g., symptoms, clinical findings, laboratory values).

n. *Misclassification* is incorrect categorization (or labeling) of the status of subjects with regard to a study variable (risk factor) that leads to a distorted (not valid or real) conclusion.

o. An *outbreak,* or *epidemic,* is a dramatic, sudden increase in a symptom, condition or health problem that is above the usual or expected rate of occurrence of the problem in a population.

p. *Attack rate* is the proportion of people in a population who develop a particular condition during an outbreak (specified time period). This proportion is sometimes called *crude attack rate.*

$$AR = \frac{\text{number of new cases (per unit of time with condition)}}{\text{number of people at risk (exposed)}}$$

q. *Food-specific attack rate* is the proportion of people in the population who develop a condition after eating a specific food.

$$AR_{ate} = \frac{\text{number of people who ate specific food and became sick}}{\text{number of people who ate specific food}}$$

$$AR_{note\ at} = \frac{\text{number of people who did not eat specific food and became sick}}{\text{number of people who did not eat specific food}}$$

r. *Secondary attack rate* is a measure of the degree of spread of a disease within a group that has been exposed to a causative agent by contact with a case.

$$Sec.\ AR = \frac{\text{number of exposed people developing disease within incubation period (specified time)}}{\text{total number of people exposed to primary case}}$$

5. The answer is b. The statement is false.

6. a. The answer is c, misclassification.

b. The answer is b. Consider the following example. In the first example (see Table AK-1), of mothers with low birth weight babies 65% stated they were smokers, and 35% stated they were nonsmokers. Meanwhile, of mothers with high birth weight babies, 20% stated they were smokers, and 80% indicated they were nonsmokers.

$$\text{Risk (odds ratio)} = \frac{65 \times 80}{20 \times 35} = \frac{5200}{700} = 7.4$$

TABLE AK-1. **True Responses**

Mothers	Low Birth Weight Baby	High Birth Weight Baby
Smoker	65	20
Nonsmoker	35	80

In the second example (see Table AK-2), of mothers with low birth weight babies, 40% stated they were smokers, and 60% stated they were nonsmokers. Meanwhile, of mothers with high birth weight babies, 20% stated they were smokers, and 80% indicated they were nonsmokers.

$$\text{Risk (odds ratio)} = \frac{40 \times 80}{20 \times 60} = \frac{3200}{1200} = 2.7$$

In the first example (Table AK-1), mothers of both low birth weight and high birth weight babies correctly reported whether they were smokers. The risk (odds ratio) of having a low birth weight baby if the mother smoked is calculated as 7.4, almost a 7.5 times greater risk for the smoking mothers.

In the second example (Table AK-2), some mothers who smoked incorrectly reported that they were not smokers. (They tended to underreport.) Approximately 38% of the smoking mothers with low birth weight babies reported that they did not smoke. Mothers with high birth weight babies correctly reported their smoking behaviors. As a result, the risk of having a low birth weight baby if the mothers' smoking status is positive is calculated as 2.7, about a 2.5 times greater risk for the smoking mothers. This measure of risk (2.7) is 64% smaller than the true risk (7.4). Thus the level of risk is deflated, or lower than it actually is.

TABLE AK-2. **Misclassification of Responses**

Mothers	Low Birth Weight Baby	High Birth Weight Baby
Smoker	40	20
Nonsmoker	60	80

7. Period prevalence is related to both point prevalence and incidence. For example, the period prevalence for a 1-year time period is equal to the point prevalence (on the first day of the year) plus the annual incidence (for that same 1-year period). Prevalence varies in direct relation to both incidence and duration. In many instances, prevalence is equal to the incidence multiplied by the average duration of the condition.

8. Several factors can affect disease prevalence in a population. As a new disease develops in a population and as new cases arise, the incidence increases. As the incidence increases, prevalence also increases. The duration of a disease also affects prevalence. When a disease has a longer duration, prevalence remains higher for a longer period. Intervention and treatment also have an impact on prevalence. As treatment reduces the number of cases, the duration of the disease and the number of cases will decrease—thus prevalence decreases.

9. Incidence rates are used to study new cases of a disease, so only the individuals at risk for developing the disease should be included in the denominator. The denominator should not include individuals who already have the disease, those who have had the disease and are no longer susceptible, or those who are not susceptible due to intervention, such as immunization.

10. a. $P_{initial} = \dfrac{117}{1275} \times \left(\dfrac{100}{100}\right) = 9.2\%$

b. $I_{10\text{-year risk}} = \dfrac{59}{1275 - 117} = \dfrac{59}{1158} \times \left(\dfrac{100}{100}\right) = 5.1\%$

11. There were 2194 users of the new OC and 12,161 nonusers. During 1998, there were 28 new cases of *Candida vaginitis* in the user population and 53 cases in the nonuser population. The incidence rate (per 1000) is calculated as follows:

$$I_{OC\text{ users}} = \dfrac{28}{2,194} \times \left(\dfrac{1000}{1000}\right) = \dfrac{12.8 \text{ cases}}{1000 \text{ users}}$$

$$I_{OC\text{ nonusers}} = \dfrac{53}{12,161} \times \left(\dfrac{1000}{1000}\right) = \dfrac{4.36 \text{ cases}}{1000 \text{ nonusers}}$$

OC users had an almost 3 times greater risk than nonusers (Risk Ratio = 12.8/4.36 = 2.9) for developing a *Candida vaginitis* infection.

12. a. Calculate the attack rate as follows:

$$AR = \dfrac{30}{600} \times \left(\dfrac{100}{100}\right) = 5\% \text{ for the 8-hour shift (time unit).}$$

b. Calculate the gender-specific attack rates as follows:

$$AR_{females} = \frac{20}{350} \times \left(\frac{100}{100}\right) = 5.7\%$$

$$AR_{males} = \frac{10}{250} \times \left(\frac{100}{100}\right) = 4\%$$

Risk Ratio (females to males) $= \dfrac{5.7}{4.0} = 1.4$ greater risk for females

c. Calculate the survey-based attack rate as follows:

$$AR = \frac{80}{400} \times \left(\frac{100}{100}\right) = 20\%$$

Attack rate should be calculated based on the number of returned survey questionnaires, not the total number of people who were sent surveys.

d. Both rates can be reported. The attack rate based on people reporting to a health facility will provide a conservative estimate (at the lower end of the range of possible values) of the outbreak, whereas the attack rate based on responses to a survey or interview will provide a liberal estimate (at the upper end of the range) of the extent of the outbreak. It should be remembered that only 70% of the healthy employees returned their survey forms, which could introduce a bias into the final results. For instance, if a large number of the nonresponding employees had experienced symptoms but did not report them through the survey, then they would not be counted among the cases, thus altering the final result determined by the study.

Chapter 3

1. The answer is c, open cohort study.

2. The answer is b. The likely effect is to decrease the apparent protective effect of exercise.

3. Match the epidemiological method with its corresponding description:

  _d_ Case series study—a collection of separate reports on individual patients used to identify a potential problem.

  _c_ Cross-sectional study—a prevalence study designed to assess the occurrence of a condition or disease.

  _e_ Case-control study—a retrospective study designed to determine causes of a disease.

_a_ Cohort study—an incidence study designed to assess attributes (variables) in a population and their relationship to the development of a condition or disease.

_b_ Clinical trial—an experimental design used to test the effectiveness of new treatments.

4. Definitions

a. A *descriptive study* attempts to uncover and portray the occurrence of the condition. Descriptive studies provide insight, data, and information on the course or patterns of disease in a population or group. Descriptive studies include case reports, case series, cross-sectional surveys, and analyses of data collected routinely over time through various databases.

b. A *case report* is a descriptive study of an individual. It reports an unusual medical occurrence, identifies a new disease, or describes adverse effects from exposure.

c. *Sampling* is the process of identifying and selecting subjects to be participants in a study. If sufficient attention is not paid to sampling, systematic error can arise in subject selection. Sampling involves drawing a smaller group of people from a larger population or group.

d. *Case selection* is the first step in a case-control study, a step that also determines the source population. In some situations, complete identification of cases in a well-defined source population may be too time consuming or otherwise impossible. Identification and collection of cases involves specifying the criteria for definition of a person as a case—in other words, as having the disease. These criteria are for inclusion in the study (eligibility criteria) as well as for exclusion from the study. Cases are found through registries, health care systems, and other sources that identify new incidence cases.

e. *Matching* is a popular approach to control for confounding in case-control studies. Its popularity reflects the notion that matching cases and controls forces these groups to be similar with respect to important risk factors, thereby making case-control comparisons less subject to confounding. The first step in matching is to identify a case. One or more potential controls, with the same or very similar values for each matching factor as the case, are then selected from the source population. For instance, matching may be made on gender and age group. More than one control can be matched with each case.

f. *Midpoint analysis* is used in cohort studies to determine whether to stop or continue the study. At a defined point in time in the study, all data collected to that point are analyzed, and a decision is made.

g. *Loss to follow-up* occurs when subjects are followed or monitored over a long period of time (in a cohort study or clinical trial). A subject may move away early or may leave the study for other reasons, including death from a cause other than the disease under investigation. If losses to follow-up are significant during the study, the validity of the results can be seriously affected.

5.   **a.** *Observational epidemiology* provides information about disease patterns by various characteristics of person, place, and time. It is used in public health for efficient allocation of resources and targeting populations for educational and prevention programs. Epidemiologists use it to generate hypotheses regarding the causes of disease or drug use problems. Investigators in observational studies may plan and identify variables to be measured, but human intervention does not take place in the process. *Analytical epidemiology* is used to test cause–effect relationships. Experimental studies involve intervention into ongoing processes to study potential changes. Some researchers do not consider experimental studies to be true epidemiological studies in the traditional sense. They are clinical or planned research designs.

b. Epidemiological studies may be retrospective or prospective in nature. In *retrospective* studies, data were collected and recorded before the study was conceived and started. In retrospective study designs, both the exposure (risk factor) and outcome (disease) occurred before the investigator initiated the study. In *prospective* studies, the planned collection of data occurs after the study has started. In these studies, outcomes have not yet occurred and exposures may have occurred before, or may be occurring during, the study period initiated by the investigator.

6.   The correct answer to the first question is C, 0.15, or 15%.

$$\text{Fall Rate (vitamin A)} = \frac{20}{400} \times 100 = 5\%$$

$$\text{Fall Rate (no vitamin A)} = \frac{80}{400} \times 100 = 20\%$$

The attributable risk difference is

$$\text{ARD} = 20\% - 5\% = 15\% \text{ (or 0.15)}.$$

The correct answer to the second question is e, 75%.

$$\text{ARF} = \frac{20\% - 5\%}{20\%} = \frac{15\%}{20\%} \times \left(\frac{100}{100}\right) = 75\%$$

7.   Calculation of incidence rate (per 1000) of photosensitivity rash in each group and the relative risk of developing rash if the new antibiotic product was being used are as follows:

$$I_{drug} = \frac{28}{2,194} \times \left(\frac{1000}{1000}\right) = \frac{12.8}{1000}$$

$$I_{no\ drug} = \frac{53}{12,161} \times \left(\frac{1000}{1000}\right) = \frac{4.4}{1000}$$

$$RR = \frac{12.8}{4.4} = 2.9$$

There is an almost 3 times greater risk of having a photosensitivity reaction if a person had used the new antibiotic.

8. Calculation of the risk of breast cancer in each group and the relative risk of developing breast cancer if a woman uses estrogens is as follows:

$$I_{estrogen\ users} = \frac{212}{4555} = 4.65\% \text{ per 15 years}$$

$$I_{nonusers} = \frac{298}{4495} = 6.63\% \text{ per 15 years}$$

$$RR = \frac{4.65}{6.63} = 0.70$$

Estrogen use provides protection against development of breast cancer.

9. Calculation of the answer is shown in Table AK-3. First, note that the data presented in the study question were incomplete with regard to constructing a 2 × 2 table or calculating an odds ratio. To perform these tasks and arrive at the answer, first calculate how many women in each age group were not using OCs according to their disease status (see third row in each age group for those numbers). For example, the number of women ages 25–29 with an MI who used OCs was 2, and the total number was 7, so the remaining amount (5) is the number of women with an MI who did not use OCs. Once this information has been derived, calculation of 6 odds ratios will identify the age group at greatest risk, if any.

Six odds ratios are calculated in this example—1 overall OR for all age groups combined and 1 OR for each age group.

$$OR_{all\ ages} = \frac{36 \times 1331}{521 \times 58} = \frac{47,916}{30,218} = 1.59$$

$$OR_{25-29} = \frac{2 \times 248}{108 \times 5} = \frac{496}{540} = 0.92$$

$$OR_{30-34} = \frac{4 \times 252}{119 \times 7} = \frac{1008}{833} = 1.21$$

TABLE AK-3. Data on Myocardial Infarction and Use of Oral Contraceptives

Age Group (years)	Exposure	Disease Status	
		MI	No Disease
25–29	Total number of women	7	356
	Number of women using OCs	2	108
	Number of women not using OCs	5	248
30–34	Total number of women	11	371
	Number of women using OCs	4	119
	Number of women not using OCs	7	252
35–39	Total number of women	9	306
	Number of women using OCs	3	85
	Number of women not using OCs	6	221
40–44	Total number of women	26	396
	Number of women using OCs	9	97
	Number of women not using OCs	17	299
45–49	Total number of women	41	423
	Number of women using OCs	18	112
	Number of women not using OCs	23	311
All ages	Total number of women	94	1852
	Number of women using OCs	31	521
	Number of women not using OCs	63	1331

Note: MI = myocardial infarction; OC = oral contraceptive.

$$OR_{35-39} = \frac{3 \times 221}{85 \times 6} = \frac{663}{510} = 1.30$$

$$OR_{40-44} = \frac{9 \times 299}{97 \times 17} = \frac{2691}{1649} = 1.63$$

$$OR_{45-49} = \frac{18 \times 311}{112 \times 23} = \frac{5598}{2576} = 2.17$$

It appears that the 40 through 44 and 45 through 49 age groups are at greatest risk, with the 45 through 49 group having the greatest risk.

Limitations of the case-control method include (1) cases and controls are not representative of the whole population, (2) there is no direct measure of incidence or prevalence, (3) recall can be biased, (4) problems can occur with exclusion criteria, (5) it can be difficult to determine that the exposure precedes the disease, and (6) this method is prone to bias in selection information.

10. The answer is calculated here based on Table AK-4.

$$OR_{alcohol} = \frac{11 \times 21}{3 \times 33} = \frac{231}{99} = 2.3$$

$$OR_{cocaine} = \frac{14 \times 45}{5 \times 23} = \frac{630}{115} = 5.5$$

Both alcohol and cocaine use increase the risk of committing suicide by Russian roulette, with cocaine use greatly increasing the risk (5.5 times greater).

Although case-control studies are easy and inexpensive to perform, they involve a small number of cases, and there can be a great loss of cases to inclusion or exclusion criteria, and how these criteria were defined (in this case, the occurrence of witnesses to verify a suicide). There also can be misclassification due to selection and recall biases. In this case, because Russian roulette is a rare event, the choice of a case-control method was appropriate. The temporal order between the attribute or exposure and disease event or health outcome can be problematic but, in this case, it is obvious. Finally, there could have been errors in blood measurement of drugs.

TABLE AK-4. Alcohol and Cocaine Use and Risk of Suicide

	Suicide by Russian Roulette	Other Drug-Related Deaths	Totals
Alcohol present	11	33	44
Alcohol absent	3	21	24
Totals	14	54	68
Cocaine present	14	23	37
Cocaine absent	5	45	50
Totals	19	68	87

Chapter 4

1. The correct answer is c, intention-to-treat analysis.

2. The correct answer is d, to obtain treatment groups with similar baseline characteristics.

3. The statement is false, not all randomized, controlled trials use placebo groups.

4. Definitions

a. *Experimental design* is a study that compares benefits of an intervention with standard treatments, or no treatment, such as a new drug therapy or prevention program, or to show cause and effect. This type of study is performed prospectively.

b. A *community intervention study* is a variation on the experimental design, in which groups of people, such as whole communities, are the unit of analysis.

c. There are many different types of contemporary *clinical trials* that use a variety of methods. The basic idea is to "try out" (trial) a new drug in clinical practice on sick patients. The goal of these clinical trials is to determine the therapeutic benefits of the new treatment. It is an experimental type of study used to determine the clinical value of a new treatment or procedure.

d. A *randomized, controlled clinical trial* refers to an experimental design that includes the randomization of subjects or patients to study groups and the use of control groups in conducting a clinical trial.

e. *Randomization* is a key aspect of clinical trials. It is the method by which patients are assigned to treatment groups to maximize the probability of the two groups being as similar as possible in terms of given background characteristics, especially background factors and variables that may influence the response to therapy or the primary outcome measure.

f. *Blinding,* or masking, is a process of keeping individulas involved in the study unaware of assignment of subjects to different study groups. Single-blind means keeping the subjects unaware; double-blind means keeping the investigators and subjects uaware; and there is even a triple-blind study, in which data analysis is done by outside evaluators independent of the investigators.

g. *Sample size determination* refers to the number of subjects who should be enrolled and the process of enrolling them in a clinical trial. The sample size should be determined soon after the primary research question or outcome has been formulated.

TABLE AK-5. **Data on Aspirin's Effectiveness in Preventing Recurrent MI**

Outcome	Aspirin Group (%)	Placebo Group (%)	Relative Risk (%)
Total mortality rate	10.8	9.7	1.12
Coronary mortality rate	8.7	8.0	1.09
Cardiovascular mortality rate	0.6	0.7	0.86
Noncardiovascular mortality rate	1.4	0.9	1.56
Mortality rate, men over 175 pounds	11.0	9.6	1.15
Mortality rate, women under 144 pounds	7.6	4.3	1.77
Mortality rate, women over 144 pounds	8.3	6.1	1.36

5. To calculate attack rates, or rates of asthma attacks, in each group:

$$AR_{\text{new drug}} = \frac{9}{29} \times \left(\frac{100}{100}\right) = 31\% \text{ (continue to have attacks)}$$

$$AR_{\text{breathing}} = \frac{12}{74} \times \left(\frac{100}{100}\right) = 16\% \text{ (continue to have attacks)}$$

The risk of having an asthma attack while on the drug, compared with the breathing exercise, is RR = 31/16 = 1.94.

The risk of having an asthma attack while on the breathing exercise, compared with the drug, is RR = 16/31 = 0.52.

Breathing exercise is more effective in preventing asthma attacks than the new drug.

6. The relative risks for death and related outcomes between the aspirin and placebo groups according to different factors are presented in Table AK-5. It appears from this study's results that aspirin does not prevent or protect a person from additional MIs. In fact, for women who have had an MI, it appears that taking aspirin increases the risk of death.

Chapter 5

1.   a. There are only four categories of season: spring, summer, fall, and winter. Season is a *discrete* multichotomous variable.

b. There are only two categories: HIV positive and HIV negative. This is a *discrete* dichotomous variable.

c. Viral load is a measurement that can assume a value anywhere along a continuum from 0 (nondetectable) to infinity; it is, therefore, a *continuous* variable.

d. CPK is an enzyme measured after a suspected myocardial infarction (MI) that can assume any value along a continuum from 0 to infinity; it is a *continuous* variable.

e. Orthopnea is often measured by the number of pillows required to sleep throughout the night. Typically, orthopnea is reported on a scale ranging from 1 to 5 pillows and is, therefore, a discrete ordinal variable.

2. The number of years diagnosed with RA can be put into categories wherein each subject would fit into only one category. One example of possible categories is displayed below in Table AK-6.

3. a. $\text{mean}_{placebo} = \dfrac{5 + 7 + 6 + 9 + 12 + 8 + 10 + 11}{8} = 8.5$

$\text{mean}_{herbal} = \dfrac{4 + 6 + 5 + 7 + 7 + 5 + 9 + 8}{8} = 6.4$

b. $\text{median}_{placebo}$ = 5, 6, 7, 8, 9, 10, 11, 12, where 8 and 9 are the middle numbers. The average of $8 + 9 = 8.5$

median_{herbal} = 4, 5, 5, 6, 7, 7, 8, 9, where 6 and 7 are the middle numbers. The average of $6 + 7 = 6.5$

c. $\text{variance}_{placebo} = \dfrac{\begin{array}{c}(5 - 8.5)^2 + (7 - 8.5)^2 + (6 - 8.5)^2 \\ + (9 - 8.5)^2 + (12 - 8.5)^2 + (8 - 8.5)^2 \\ + (10 - 8.5)^2 + (11 - 8.5)^2\end{array}}{7} = 6$

TABLE AK-6. Number of Years Diagnosed with RA as a Discrete Variable

Number of Years Diagnosed with RA	Placebo	Herbal
< 5 years	0	1
5–9 years	5	7
10–14 years	3	0

$$variance_{herbal} = \frac{\begin{array}{c}(4 - 6.4)^2 + (6 - 6.4)^2 + (5 - 6.4)^2 \\ + (7 - 6.4)^2 + (7 - 6.4)^2 + (5 - 6.4)^2 \\ + (9 - 6.4)^2 + (8 - 6.4)^2\end{array}}{7} = 2.84$$

d. $SD_{placebo} = \sqrt{6} = 2.5$

$SD_{herbal} = \sqrt{2.84} = 1.7$

e. $SE_{placebo} = \dfrac{2.5}{\sqrt{8}} = 0.89$

$SE_{herbal} = \dfrac{1.6}{\sqrt{8}} = 0.60$

f. $95\% \text{ CI } \mu_{placebo} = 8.5 \pm (2.0)0.89 = (6.7, 10.3)$

$95\% \text{ CI } \mu_{herbal} = 6.4 \pm (2.0)0.60 = (5.2, 7.6)$

4. The data are continuous, and the sample size is less than 30. The data are also unpaired. If the data are normally distributed, then the t-test is appropriate.

5. The data in Table 5-10 can be statistically analyzed using the t-test as follows:

  a. State the null hypothesis to be tested via the t-test.

  H_0: mean years diagnosed with $RA_{placebo}$ = mean years diagnosed with RA_{herbal} or

  H_0: mean years diagnosed with $RA_{placebo}$ − mean years diagnosed with RA_{herbal} = 0

  b. Calculate the means and variances for each group.

$$mean_{placebo} = 8.5 \quad mean_{herbal} = 6.4$$
$$variance_{placebo} = 6$$
$$variance_{herbal} = 2.84$$

  c. Calculate the pooled variance.

$$S_p^2 = \frac{(n_1 - 1)s_1^2 + (n_2 - 1)s_2^2}{n_1 + n_2 - 2}$$

$$S_p^2 = \frac{(8 - 1)6 + (8 - 1)2.84}{8 + 8 - 2}$$

$$S_p^2 = 4.42$$

d. Calculate the t-value.

$$t = \frac{\mu_1 - \mu_2}{SE\,(\mu_1 - \mu_2)}$$

where $SE\,(\mu_1 - \mu_2) = S_p^2 \sqrt{\dfrac{1}{n_1} + \dfrac{1}{n_2}}$

$$t = \frac{8.5 - 6.4}{4.42\sqrt{\frac{1}{8} + \frac{1}{8}}}$$

$$t = 0.950$$

e. Use a t-value distribution table (see Appendix II) to determine the critical value of t. The degrees of freedom for the t-test are as follows:

$$df = n_1 + n_2 - 2$$

$$df = 8 + 8 - 2 = 14$$

Appendix II shows that for degrees of freedom $= 14$, the critical t-value required to reject the null hypothesis is 2.145. Therefore, any calculated t-value greater than 2.145 or less than -2.145, will lead to rejection of the null hypothesis. In this example, the calculated value of t is 0.950. This calculated t-value is less than 2.145 and greater than -2.145, the critical values of t; therefore, the null hypothesis is accepted.

f. Interpret and report the results of the analysis.

The mean years diagnosed with RA in the placebo group is not statistically different from the mean years diagnosed with RA in the herbal group.

6. Degree of pain is a discrete, or ordinal, variable. Degree of pain is measured on a scale of 1 through 5. There are only five categories or options for this variable.

7. Appendix I can be used to determine the appropriate statistical test to analyze the data. Degree of pain at the end of the study is unpaired, discrete data. If 75% or more of the expected cells are ≥ 5, then the Chi-Square Test can be used. If $<75\%$ of the expected cells are ≥ 5, the Fisher's Exact Test can be used.

8. The degree of pain relief is determined by subtracting the degree of pain at the end of the study from the degree of pain at baseline. This involves analyzing two measurements per subject; therefore, degree of pain in this example is considered to be paired data. Therefore, the McNemar's Test is appropriate to analyze the data.

TABLE AK-7. **Observed Herbal Use in a Study**

	Yes	No	Total
Male	125	375	500
Female	238	462	700
	363	837	1200

9. The Chi-Square Test is most appropriate

a. H_0: Proportion of herbal use males = Proportion of herbal use females

b. Plot the observed frequencies in a 2×2 contingency table. The observed frequencies are plotted in Table AK-7.

c. Calculate the corresponding expected frequency for each cell. The expected frequencies are shown in Table AK-8.

d. Count the number of expected cells with frequencies equal to or less than 5. None of the expected frequencies is less than or equal to 5; therefore, the Chi-Square Test is appropriate to use for this sample.

e. Calculate a Chi-Square value.

$$X^2 = \Sigma \left\{ \frac{(O - E)^2}{E} \right\}$$

$$X^2 = \frac{(125 - 151)^2}{51} + \frac{(375 - 349)^2}{349} + \frac{(238 - 212)^2}{212} + \frac{(462 - 489)^2}{489}$$

$$= 11.12$$

TABLE AK-8. **Expected Gender Frequencies in a Study**

	Yes	No	Total
Male	$\frac{(125 + 375)(125 + 238)}{1200} = 151$	$\frac{(125 + 375)(375 + 462)}{1200} = 349$	500
Female	$\frac{(238 + 462)(125 + 238)}{1200} = 212$	$\frac{(238 + 462)(375 + 462)}{1200} = 489$	700
	363	837	1200

f. Use a Chi-Square distribution table (see Appendix III) to determine the critical X^2 value required to reject the null hypothesis for the degrees of freedom calculated from the sample. The calculated X^2 value is 11.12, with degrees of freedom = $(R - 1)(C - 1)$ degrees of freedom = $(2 - 1)(2 - 1) = 1$. The X^2 critical value required to reject the null hypothesis at $p = 0.05$ for degrees of freedom = 1 is 3.84. Because the calculated X^2 value (11.12) is greater than the X^2 critical value (3.84), the null hypothesis is rejected.

g. Interpret and report the results of the analysis:

The proportion of females who used herbal medications in the past year is statistically different from the proportion of men who used herbal medications in the past year.

Chapter 6

1. Definitions

a. *Cumulative incidence*—the number of new cases of cancer for a 1-year period.

b. *Prevalence*—the number of existing cases of hepatatoxicity among HIV-positive subjects at a specific point in time. Remember, only prevalence can be obtained from a cross-sectional study because both exposure and outcome are measured simultaneously.

c. *Cumulative incidence*—the number of new cases of nonfatal firearm-related injuries during a 1-year period.

d. *Incidence* (mortality rate)—the number of cases of death among all firearm-related injuries during a 1-year period.

e. *Incidence rate*—the number of new cases of cough among ACE-inhibitor users for a given time period of observation. Note that the units are in person-time.

2. **a.** This is an example of a case-control study. Subjects are chosen based on outcome status (MI or no MI) and then exposure (CAD) is measured and compared.

b. Because this is a case-control design, the odds ratio is the most appropriate risk estimate to use. Subjects are first plotted into a 2 × 2 contingency table as shown in Table AK-9.

$$OR = \frac{AD}{BC}$$

$$OR = \frac{(100)(680)}{(900)(20)}$$

TABLE AK-9. **2 × 2 Contingency Table for CAD and MI**

CORONARY ARTERY DISEASE (CAD)	MYOCARDIAL INFARCTION		
	Yes	No	Total
Yes	100	900	1000
No	20	680	700
Total	120	1580	1700

$$OR = \frac{68,000}{18,000}$$

$$OR = 3.8$$

Subjects with CAD are 3.8 times more likely to have an MI than subjects without CAD.

c. The 95% confidence interval are calculated as follows:

$$95\% \text{ CI OR} = OR e^{\pm z\sqrt{1/a+1/b+1/c+1/d}} \quad \text{or}$$

$$95\% \text{ CI} = (ad/bc)e^{\pm z\sqrt{1/a+1/b+1/c+1/d}}$$

$$95\% \text{ CI} = 3.8e^{\pm 1.96\sqrt{1/100+1/900+1/20+1/680}}$$

$$95\% \text{ CI} = 3.8e^{\pm 0.49}$$

$$95\% \text{ CI} = (2.3, 6.2)$$

d. Yes, the risk estimate is statistically significant. The null hypothesis is **not** included within the bounds of the 95% confidence interval; therefore, the result is statistically significant and would result in a p-value ≤ 0.05. Because this example measures the odds ratio, the null hypothesis states that the $OR = 1$. Because the number 1 is not included within the bounds of the cumulative incidence (3.6, 4.15), the results are statistically significant.

e. Given the narrow width of the 95% confidence interval, this calculation appears to generate a reliable risk estimate. This is predominantly a function of the large sample size.

f. There are many potentional confounders, including age, gender, race, diet, exercise, positive family history of CAD or heart disease, and smoking.

3. **a.** RR = 1.36. This represents an increased risk. Therefore, the excess risk 36% (0.36) is added on to the null hypothesis (1.0).

b. RR = 0.69. The reduction in risk is 31% (0.31). Therefore, the decreased risk (0.31) is subtracted from the null hypothesis (1.0).

Chapter 7

1. Definitions

a. *Validity* refers to the degree to which a measure actually measures what it is designed to measure. Internal validity is the extent to which the results of a study accurately reflect the situation in reality, whereas external validity is the extent to which the study's results are applicable to other populations.

b. *Reliability* is the degree of stability exhibited when a measurement is repeated under identical conditions. Reliability refers to the degree to which a measure or result can be replicated. Lack of reliability may arise from divergence among observers or instruments of measurement or from the instability of the attribute being measured. Reliability may be thought of as reproducibility or repeatability; it is not a guarantee of validity.

c. *Bias* is systematic error in a study that leads to distortion of the results so that the results do not accurately reflect reality. Bias can result during the selection of a study sample or during information and data collection, or it can result from the influence of a confounding variable.

d. A *confounding variable* influences the relationship between an independent variable (e.g., exposure, risk factor) and a dependent variable (e.g., disease, study outcome), altering the true relationship between them. A potential confounding variable must be associated with the disease or outcome of interest in the absence of the exposure, and it must be associated with the exposure but not as a consequence of the exposure. Potential confounding variables are usually limited to established risk factors of the disease under study.

e. A *screening test* is used to identify people suspected of having a disease. If there is a positive result, then the person can be given more definitive diagnostic studies and examination. The purpose of screening populations is to detect as many people with a disease (cases) as possible. Screening and disease detection are very important aspects of public health. Screening programs are one tool used to meet the need of preventing disease in a population. Screening can be defined as the use of quick and simple testing procedures to identify and separate people who are apparently well but who may be at risk for a disease from those who probably do not have the disease.

f. *Sensitivity* is the probability that a person who actually has the condition will have a positive (abnormal) test result.

$$\text{Sen} = \frac{\text{number of people with disease who test positive}}{\begin{array}{c}\text{number of people with disease who test positive}\\ + \text{ number of people with disease who test negative}\end{array}}$$

g. *Specificity* is the probability that a person who actually does not have the condition will have a negative (normal) test result.

$$\text{SPE} = \frac{\text{number of people without disease who test negative}}{\begin{array}{c}\text{number of people without disease who test negative}\\ + \text{ number of people without disease who test positive}\end{array}}$$

h. *Positive predictive value* is the probability that a person with a positive (abnormal) test result actually has the disease under study.

$$\text{PV+} = \frac{\text{number of people with disease who test positive}}{\begin{array}{c}\text{number of people with disease who test positive}\\ + \text{ number of people without disease who test positive}\end{array}}$$

i. *Negative predictive value* is the probability that a person with a negative (normal) test result actually does not have the disease.

$$\text{PV-} = \frac{\text{number of people without disease who test negative}}{\begin{array}{c}\text{number of people without disease who test negative}\\ + \text{ number of people with disease who test negative}\end{array}}$$

2. There is a relationship between sensitivity and specificity in terms of setting the cutoff point, or the limit for a normal test result. A test can have a range of values, and it becomes important to decide where the cutoff for positive versus negative test results will be set. With the choice of one value, the test will correctly identify most of the sick people in a population (true positives), but it will miss a small proportion of the sick subjects in a population (false negatives). In contrast, the test will not identify most of the healthy people as having the disease (true negatives), but it will indicate that a few healthy people have the disease (false positives). Moving the cutoff limit of the test's value down to a lower number in its range will change the results. In this situation, the test will correctly identify all of the sick people in a population but at a cost. More healthy people will be identified as having the disease when, in reality, they do not. Moving the cutoff number down has increased the test's sensitivity, but it also decreased its specificity. The cutoff limit of the test's value also could be moved up to a higher number in its range. Although none of the healthy people would then be identified as having the disease, many

TABLE AK-10. **Value of Hair Test for Cocaine Use**

Hair Test	Cocaine-Positive Blood Test	Cocaine-Negative Blood Test	Totals
Positive	475 (A)	475 (B)	950
Negative	25 (C)	9025 (D)	9050
Totals	500	9500	10,000

more sick people would be missed by the test, showing negative results (a normal test value). Moving the cutoff number up increased the test's specificity, but it also decreased its sensitivity. Determining the best cutoff level, or limit, for a screening test is one of the most important considerations in planning and performing a screening program.

3. The predictive value of a screening test is determined by its validity and by characteristics of the population being tested, especially the prevalence of preclinical disease. The higher the prevalence of a disease in a population, the more the sensitivity and the specificity of a test affects its predictive value. The higher the prevalence of a disease in a population, the more likely it is that higher numbers of true positives will occur. The more sensitive the test and the higher the predictive value, then the lower the numbers of false positives.

4. The results of both the hair test and a blood test for the presence of cocaine in these 10,000 people are presented in Table AK-10. The value of the new hair test is determined by calculating its sensitivity and specificity.

$$\text{Sen} = \frac{475}{475 + 25} = \frac{475}{500} = 0.95, \text{ or } 95\%$$

$$\text{SPE} = \frac{9025}{9025 + 475} = \frac{9025}{9500} = 0.95, \text{ or } 95\%$$

The hair test for cocaine use has 95% sensitivity and 95% specificity.

Chapter 8

1. *Postmarketing surveillance* is defined as the monitoring of the uses and effects of drugs after they are approved by the FDA. Because premarketing studies involve phase I, II, and III trials, studies conducted after marketing are sometimes referred to as *phase IV trials*.

2. There are several limitations of premarketing trials for detection of adverse drug reactions. Premarketing randomized clinical trials are short in duration and cannot assess long-term effects of drugs. Premarketing randomized clinical trials also have specific inclusion and exclusion criteria that result in studies on homogenous populations. This experience may not be reflective of who will use the drug after FDA approval. Drugs are studied for a single indication; however, once the drug is released, it will be used for many unapproved indications. Finally, premarketing randomized clinical trials cannot detect rare adverse drug reactions.

3. Methods used to monitor drugs after FDA approval include descriptive methods (e.g., spontaneous reporting systems, case reports and series, cross-sectional studies), observational studies (e.g., cohort and case-control studies), interventional studies, and meta-analyses.

4. Adverse drug reactions are underreported in the United States. Therefore, the number of subjects experiencing a particular adverse drug reaction is unknown. Because information on the number of subjects exposed to a particular drug is unavailable, it is not possible to determine the incidence of an adverse drug reaction. In addition, information about confounding variables is often incomplete or inaccurate. Spontaneous reports are subject to bias and are highest when the drug is newly released onto the market. Finally, there is no comparison group.

5. The FDA can force the manufacturer to update the drug label, or package insert, to include information about the adverse drug reaction. The FDA can mandate that the manufacturer distribute letters to health care professionals informing them about the adverse drug reaction, or it can require formal surveillance of the drug. The FDA can also recommend withdrawal of the drug from the market.

Chapter 9

1. *Pharmacoeconomics* is the area of health care research that evaluates and compares the costs and outcomes associated with drug therapy.

2. Pharmacoeconomical research differ from clinical trials in the following ways: As compared to clinical trial research pharmacoeconomical outcome research is concerned with evaluating the drug in the "real world." The primary role of clinical trials is to measure the efficacy and safety of a drug. In contrast, pharmacoeconomical research attempts to measure the efficacy of the drug or its overall value in the health care system. It not only evaluates drug therapy outcomes but also compares and contrasts these outcomes in terms of their cost. Another fundamental difference between pharmacoeconomical research and clinical trial research is how the results may be extrapolated. In general, the results of a well-designed clinical study conducted in one country are also applicable to other countries. However, given the differences in monetary exchange rates and cultures across countries, the same cannot be said of pharmacoeconomical studies.

3. Definitions

a. *Clinical outcomes* include the results of treatment with a drug and may be both favorable (e.g., curing, preventing, or slowing the progression of a disease) and unfavorable (e.g., toxicity).

b. *Humanistic outcomes* look at the patients' point of view and address such questions as how the patient feels and how he or she perceives quality of life.

c. *Direct medical costs* are associated with the drug and the medical care itself and include acquisition costs, monitoring costs, preparation costs and physicians' fees, costs of administrating the medication (e.g., IV administration sets, infusion pumps), as well as the cost of treating an adverse drug reaction.

d. *Direct nonmedical costs* are relevant to providing therapy and include transportation to a health care facility and ancillary support, such as social and home care services.

e. *Indirect costs* result from a loss of productivity (e.g., loss of income, days of school missed) due to illness. These costs are associated with the morbidity and mortality of a disease.

f. *Intangible costs* are costs associated with pain and suffering of disease and may greatly affect a patient's well-being and quality of life. These costs are difficult to which to assign a dollar value.

g. *Discounting* is the process of adjusting future costs and discounting them back to their present value. The premise behind discounting is that a dollar now is worth more than it would be in the future.

h. The *study perspective* is the point of view from which it is conducted. A study may have different perspectives, including a hospital or other health care provider, a payer, a patient, or society in general.

4. A cost-minimization analysis is based on the assumption that the outcomes of the alternatives being assessed are equal in all respects, including efficacy and adverse reactions. The total costs of the alternatives are then compared, and the least expensive alternative is selected. If the alternatives are not equal, than a cost-minimization analysis is not valid.

5. **a.** A cost-benefit analysis measures both costs and benefits in monetary units. The benefits in this case would be any cost savings associated with the anticoagulation clinic. Therefore, the costs before the clinic was implemented should be compared to the costs after the clinic was implemented, as shown in Table 9-6. The B/C ratio would be $177,000/132,000, or 1.34/1.

b. Based on the benefit-to-cost ratio calculated, the anticoagulation clinic is cost-beneficial. For each $1 spent on the clinic, the hospital saved $1.34.

6. a. To determine the cost-effectiveness (C/E) ratio for drug A, one first calculates the costs associated with each path of the decision tree based on the cumulative probability and costs of an outcome occurring as follows:

$$\text{Cost of path 1} = (0.85)(0.70)(\$1500) = \$892.50$$

$$\text{Cost of path 2} = (0.85)(0.30)(\$2000) = \$510.00$$

$$\text{Cost of path 3} = (0.15)(0.90)(\$4000) = \$540.00$$

$$\text{Cost of path 4} = (0.15)(0.10)(\$5000) = \$\ 75.00$$

The total costs for all four paths are then calculated, and are $2017.50. The C/E ratio of drug A is equal to the total costs divided by the efficacy ($2017.50/.85), or $2373.53/treatment success.

b. The C/E ratio for drug B is calculated similarly as follows:

$$\text{Cost of path 5} = (0.65)(0.90)(\$1000) = \$585.00$$

$$\text{Cost of path 6} = (0.65)(0.10)(\$1500) = \$\ 97.50$$

$$\text{Cost of path 7} = (0.35)(0.80)(\$3000) = \$840.00$$

$$\text{Cost of path 8} = (0.35)(0.20)(\$4000) = \underline{\$280.00}$$

Total costs $1802.50

$$\text{C/E ratio} = \frac{\text{Total costs}}{\text{efficacy}} \left(\frac{\$1802.50}{0.65}\right) = \frac{\$2773}{\text{treatment success}}$$

c. Drug A costs $2373.53/treatment success, and drug B costs $2773/treatment success. Therefore, drug A would be more cost-effective.

7. We would calculate the C/E ratio for drug B with a probability for success as 0.80 and probability for failure as 0.20. The C/E ratio for drug B is calculated as follows:

$$\text{Cost of path 5} = (0.80)(0.90)(\$1000) = \$720$$

$$\text{Cost of path 6} = (0.80)(0.10)(\$1500) = \$120$$

$$\text{Cost of path 7} = (0.20)(0.80)(\$3000) = \$480$$

$$\text{Cost of path 8} = (0.20)(0.20)(\$4000) = \underline{\$160}$$

Total costs $1480

$$\text{C/E ratio} = \frac{\text{Total costs}}{\text{efficacy}} \left(\frac{\$1480}{0.80}\right) = \frac{\$1850}{\text{treatment success}}$$

Based on a different probability for success, drug B is more cost-effective, which illustrates why a sensitivity analysis should be performed to test results under various assumptions.

8. The incremental cost effectiveness (ICE) ratio is calculated by comparing the differences in costs and outcomes of two therapies as follows:

$$\text{ICE ratio} = \frac{(\text{cost therapy B} - \text{cost therapy A})}{(\text{success therapy A} - \text{success therapy B})}$$

$$\text{ICE ratio} = \frac{(\$2000 - \$1800)}{(0.90 - 0.70)} = \frac{\$200}{0.2} = \frac{\$1000}{\text{treatment success}}.$$

The ICE ratio represents the additional cost to the organization if Therapy B is selected as the preferred alternative.

9. **a.** To calculate QALYs for drug A, one multiplies the quality of life utility (0.80) times the life expectancy for the patient (6 years). The QALYs would be 4.8.

b. To calculate QALYs for drug B, one multiplies the quality of life utility (0.90) times the life expectancy for the patient (5 years). The QALYs would be 4.5.

c. The incremental cost-utility (ICU) ratio of therapy A can be calculated as described in question 8 except with a CUA, success is measured in QALYs.

$$\text{ICU ratio} = \frac{(\text{costs therapy B} - \text{cost therapy A})}{(\text{QALYs therapy A} - \text{QALYs therapy B})}$$

Therefore, in this case the

$$\text{ICU ratio} = \frac{(\$30,000 - \$15,000)}{(4.8 - 4.5)} = \left(\frac{\$15,000}{0.3}\right)$$
$$= \$30,000 \text{ per treatment success.}$$

10. **a.** The undiscounted B/C ratio is the ratio of the total costs of benefits realized by the drug (e.g., costs of hospitalizations avoided) over the 5 years to the drug costs incurred over that time.

$$\frac{B}{C} = \frac{(\text{Total benefit costs})}{(\text{Total drug costs})} = \left(\frac{\$160,000}{\$150,000}\right) = \frac{1.06}{1}$$

The new drug is slightly cost-beneficial: $1.06 saved for every dollar spent.

b. Using the discount factor in Table 9-1, the discounted costs are now as shown in Table AK-11.

The adjusted B/C ratio is now $133,500/$134,530 = 0.99/1.

TABLE AK-11.	DISCOUNTED COSTS FOR QUESTION 10

Adjusted Costs for Drug	*Adjusted Benefits Costs*
Year 1 ($50,000)(0.952) = $47,600	Year 1 ($10,000)(0.952) = $ 9,520
Year 2 ($50,000)(0.907) = $45,350	Year 2 ($10,000)(0.907) = $ 9,070
Year 3 ($20,000)(0.864) = $17,280	Year 3 ($40,000)(0.864) = $34,560
Year 4 ($20,000)(0.823) = $16,460	Year 4 ($50,000)(0.823) = $41,150
Year 5 ($10,000)(0.784) = $ 7,840	Year 5 ($50,000)(0.784) = $39,200
Total adjusted costs = $134,530	$133,500

c. Based on the 5% discount rate, the new drug would now not be considered to be cost-beneficial: $0.99 saved for every dollar spent. (See Figure AK-1.)

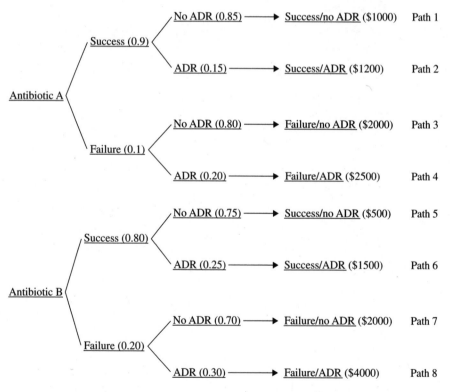

Figure AK-1. Decision tree for antibiotic therapies A and B. (ADR = adverse drug reaction.)

Figure 10-1 Decision tree for antibiotic therapies A and B. (ADR = adverse drug reaction.)

Chapter 10

1. The best decisions regarding drug therapy are decisions based on evidence. Drugs are shown to be safe and effective in the context of well-designed studies. Before clinicians make decisions about drug therapy, the medical literature should be searched for evidence. The type of study, methodology, and quality of the data all should be considered when evaluating a study. The Cochrane database offers systematic reviews of traditional and nontraditional therapies to aid the practitioner in the practice of evidence-based medicine.

2. Case-control studies are the most obvious application of institutional adverse drug reaction reporting systems. If spontaneous reports lead practitioners to believe that there is a problem with a particular drug, then a case-control study can be conducted to formally test the hypothesis. The advantage of case-control studies over spontaneous reports is the ability to identify and measure the role of confounders in the suspected reaction. The case-control study also offers a comparison group.

3. Cohort studies are the most obvious application of institutional DUEs. Data collected for DUEs are very similar to data collected in prospective cohort studies. The cohort offers the advantage of a comparison group and the ability to measure the effect of confounding variables.

4. Pharmacoeconomic methods can be applied to formulary management. Formulary considerations can include not only the cost of the drug but also the value of the drug therapy. Pharmacoeconomics can also be applied to disease-state management.

5. Instead of collecting data on individual patients, pharmacists can collect routine data on all patients. The pharmacist should first determine research and null hypotheses to be tested. Then, relevant information is collected on patients pertaining to demographics, past and current medical history, medication history, laboratory values, and so forth. The information can be collected and stored in a database. In this regard, the patients become subjects in a cohort study.

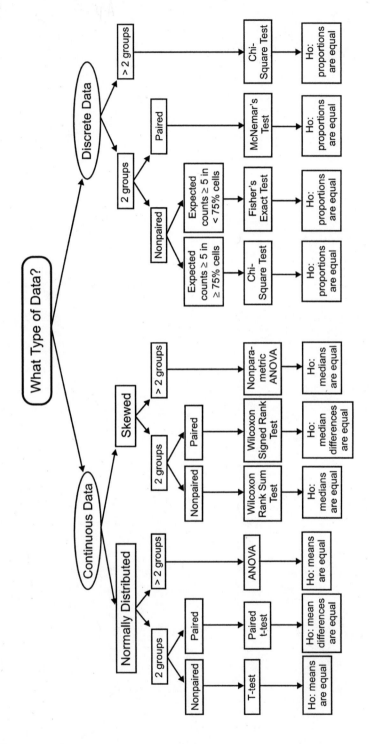

Flow chart to determine appropriate statistical test to analyze data

Critical Values of *t* Required to Reject the Null Hypothesis for a 2-Tailed Test

df	p = 0.05	p = 0.01	p = 0.001
1	12.706	63.657	636.619
2	4.303	9.925	31.598
3	3.182	5.841	12.941
4	2.776	4.604	8.610
5	2.571	4.032	6.859
6	2.447	3.707	5.959
7	2.365	3.499	5.405
8	2.306	3.355	5.041
9	2.262	3.250	4.781
10	2.228	3.169	4.587
11	2.201	3.106	4.437
12	2.179	3.055	4.318
13	2.160	3.012	4.221
14	2.145	2.977	4.140
15	2.131	2.947	4.073
16	2.120	2.921	4.015
17	2.110	2.898	3.965
18	2.101	2.818	3.922
19	2.093	2.861	3.883
20	2.086	2.845	3.850
100	1.984	2.626	3.391
infinite	1.96	2.576	3.292

Critical Values of X^2 Required to Reject the Null Hypothesis

df	0.05	0.01	0.001
1	3.84	6.64	10.83
2	5.99	9.21	13.82
3	7.82	11.34	16.27
4	9.49	13.28	18.46
5	11.07	15.09	20.52
6	12.59	16.81	22.46
7	14.07	18.48	24.32
8	15.51	20.09	26.12
9	16.92	21.67	27.88
10	18.31	23.21	29.59
11	19.68	24.72	31.26
12	21.03	26.22	32.91
13	22.36	27.69	34.53
14	23.68	29.14	36.12
15	25.00	30.58	37.70
16	26.3	32.00	39.29
17	27.59	33.41	40.75
18	28.87	34.80	42.31
19	30.14	36.19	43.82
20	31.41	37.57	45.32
21	32.67	38.93	46.80
22	33.92	40.29	48.27
23	35.17	41.64	49.73
24	36.42	42.98	51.18
25	37.65	44.31	52.62
26	38.88	45.64	54.05
27	40.11	46.96	55.48
28	41.34	48.28	56.89
29	42.56	49.59	58.30
30	43.77	50.89	59.70

INDEX